# ICD-9-CM and POA Coding Mentor

# ICD-9-CM and POA Coding Mentor

## A Learning Tool for Interpreting Health Records

PATRICIA L. BOWER-JERNIGAN, RHIA
Allina Health System

EDITOR

**HEALTH FORUM, INC.**
*An American Hospital Association Company*
Chicago

*I dedicate this book to my mom and dad,*
*who truly believed in the power*
*of furthering one's own education,*
*and to Roy, Stewart, Charles, and Liesl.*
*May your educational journey never end.*

# CONTENTS

# ABOUT THE EDITOR

PATRICIA BOWER-JERNIGAN, RHIA, is director of system-wide hospital coding for Allina's eleven hospitals, which are located in Minnesota and Wisconsin. She directs, coordinates, and facilitates hospital inpatient and outpatient coding staff to provide accurate diagnostic and procedural coding data for statistical, financial, clinical, and quality improvement processes. She also promotes the effective use of data for assessing and improving the quality of customer services and clinical outcomes.

Ms. Bower-Jernigan has more than twenty-five years' experience with coding, HIM, and consulting on health care revenue cycle improvement processes. She has also been an educator, teaching health information students in ICD-9-CM, CPT coding, and medical terminology.

Since 2007, Ms. Bower-Jernigan has served as a member of the editorial advisory board of *AHA Coding Clinic® for ICD-9-CM,* a quarterly publication of the Central Office on ICD-9-CM of the American Hospital Association. In her role as a board member, she represents hospitals in the process of developing national coding guidelines.

# CONTRIBUTORS

**LAURA CAMPBELL, MS,** has served the Allina Hospitals and Clinics since 2006, where she is a training supervisor in the Revenue Cycle Management Department. During that time, she has worked to lead training standardization and documentation process updates across the Allina system. Under her leadership, trainers collaborate throughout the system to produce high-quality revenue cycle training tools and programs for employees. In addition, her role has expanded to managing the administration of an electronic verification system. Ms. Campbell holds a master of science degree in training and organizational development and is passionate about employee education. She is an active member of training and professional organizations within the St. Paul/Minneapolis area.

**JOANN COLE, RN,** has served the Allina Hospitals since 1988. She initially worked for twelve years providing direct patient care, including as charge nurse for the orthopedic/neurology and mother/baby units. She has served Allina in her current role as an MS-DRG documentation specialist for more than eight years. In this role, she works with health care providers, including physicians, and with coding staff to ensure that the coding process is accurate and concise. She reviews records concurrently and retrospectively, providing feedback for quality improvement and training purposes. Her role was recently expanded to include the development of educational tools and resources for excellence in documentation and the presentation of education and training throughout the Allina system.

**DIANE KOURY, CCS-P,** is a coding data specialist with Allina Hospitals. She is actively involved in the Allina coding float pool to assist the eleven hospital sites with inpatient and outpatient coding. She brings eight years of experience in the hospital coding and HIM settings.

**WENDY MILLER, MD,** is an internal medicine physician at Abbott Northwestern Hospital in Minneapolis. She received her medical doctorate from the University of Minnesota and completed her residency and chief residency at Hennepin County Medical Center in Minneapolis. She currently serves as lead physician for the Abbott Northwestern Hospitalist Service.

**JANE STENHOLM, RN, BSN,** is an MS-DRG documentation specialist with Allina Hospitals. She has more than eight years' experience in the quality and HIM setting, where she has specialized in documentation needs. In her current role, she works directly with health care providers and coding staff to ensure that documentation for the coding process is accurate and concise. Her duties have included performing concurrent and retrospective chart review, creating educational tools, giving presentations for both the coding staff and health care providers, and collecting statistical data for the organization. Before moving to the quality and HIM setting, she spent twelve years in the intensive care arena as a charge nurse and direct care provider.

**TIERZA STEPHAN, MD, FACP,** is district medical director for Allina Medical Clinic Hospitalists. She has worked as a hospitalist since 1995. Her past positions include chairperson of the Department of Medicine, treasurer of the medical staff, and lead physician of Abbott Northwestern Hospitalist Service. She is a long-standing member of the peer review committee for the Department of Medicine and is the chairperson of the Graduate Medical Education Committee.

**JENNIFER THIRY, RHIT,** is an inpatient coding coordinator for all eleven Allina hospitals. She serves as a resource to Allina's coders regarding ICD-9-CM and MS-DRG coding. She brings twenty years of experience in the inpatient hospital coding arena.

**MICHELLE WRIGHT, RHIT,** is a coding data specialist with Allina Hospitals. She has nineteen years of coding experience, primarily in the inpatient hospital setting. She has been a part of the Allina coding float pool for the past four years and is a long-standing member of the Allina coding task force.

# ACKNOWLEDGMENTS

Many people have been instrumental in the development of this project, having devoted endless hours while sharing their expertise, knowledge, and professionalism. Each of these individuals was open to the vision of the project, accepted the unknown, and embraced the journey with an open mind. Thank you for being a part of the big team.

I am full of gratitude to Diane Koury, Jennifer Thiry, and Michelle Wright for sharing their coding expertise. They were proactive in identifying what was working and came up with alternatives, when needed, so the project could keep moving.

I am also thankful to Joann Cole and Jane Stenholm. You bring such value and insight into reviewing the medical documentation and have a gift for educating others in a non-threatening way. Your positive approach to work is a delight to behold, and I appreciate your honesty and the professionalism you bring to others.

I would like to express my gratitude to Wendy Miller, MD, and Tierza Stephan, MD, for their medical expertise and the time they spent reviewing diagnoses and clinical indicators for this project. You are outstanding physicians who truly understand the relationship between physician documentation and the coder's process for using that documentation to complete his or her work.

I would like to pass on a very special thank you to Laura Campbell for spending many long nights working on the layout for this project. Your creativity and ideas were welcomed and greatly appreciated throughout the whole process.

I am grateful to Joan Yohn for believing in me and supporting my professional journey during the creation of this book. You are a wonderful mentor, and it is always good to know that I am "one lucky, loopy mom."

I would also like to show my appreciation to a number of other Allina staff who assisted with this project: Ben Peltier, Jodie Mortenson, Deb Pavel, Glenyce Klaers, Barb Fleischer, Megan O'Neill, Sheri Johns, Anna Hallquist, and Terri McLean. And, of course, I cannot forget the very important HIM operations staff, who produced many copies of records for the team to review.

Finally, many thanks to my AHA Press contacts, Richard Hill, Christopher Hund, and Joyce Dunne. I appreciate your brilliant leadership in editing this book and the support you brought to me along the way.

# HOW TO USE THIS WORKBOOK

This workbook is designed to be used in many different, multipurpose ways, including the following:

- As a workbook for novice or inexperienced inpatient hospital coding staff to help advance their proficiency as coders. The workbook will strengthen the thought process behind their coding decisions, allowing them to become more independent and competent, leading to favorable results for the hospital's quality of coding collection.
- As a text for academic programs that offers actual, copied automated health records, with guidance on how to select appropriate documentation that supports the ICD-9-CM codes, along with POA and MS-DRG assignments.
- As a support tool for coding managers who wish to improve staff coding skills but may not have the one-to-one resources for mentoring effectively.
- As a source of information to guide coders in understanding clinical workflow processes and common diagnosis resource indicators, including examples of QHCP queries.

The workbook includes a compact disk with seventy-five health records. The records are organized based on the twenty-five chapters of the workbook, with three health records available for each chapter. The records are arranged in order of complexity of coding, which range from *basic* to *intermediate* to *advanced*. The coder should open the disk; select the chapter of interest; read all the documentation from the health record; and assign all the ICD-9-CM diagnoses and procedures as appropriate to the individual record, as well as POA indicators for each diagnosis. If MS-DRG grouper tools are available, the coder should also assign an MS-DRG for the health record.

If the coding manager desires, the coder may be asked to document, in the "Coding Clinic Reference/Reason" section of the answer key grids, the source of supporting documentation. The references to *Coding Clinic* in the workbook and answer key come from the pages of *AHA Coding Clinic® for ICD-9-CM*, a quarterly publication of the Central Office on ICD-9-CM of the American Hospital Association.

Appendix A, "Clinical Workflow Process Tools," contains information that may be useful when considering whether a specific diagnosis should be confirmed by the QHCP. It is important to review the clinical findings within the laboratory and radiology reports as well as the patient's described condition to determine if a more specific diagnosis can be established. It is equally important to look at the clinical findings for other common conditions often associated with that diagnosis. The use of this tool can help guide the coder to determine when a query may appropriately be initiated.

Appendix B, "Common Diagnosis Resource Indicators," is a reference to which the coder may refer for detailed descriptions of high-volume diagnoses. This appendix provides definitions and specific requirements of diagnoses, as well as the common clinical indicators that are seen with each diagnosis. Appendix B assists the coder in understanding the necessary clinical components when formulating a query, thus enabling the coder to get to the greatest specificity of a diagnosis.

Appendix C, "Qualified Health Care Professional Query Guidelines and Tools," contains information for a coder when—after reviewing the clinical findings within the laboratory and radiology reports and considering the patient's described condition—a query to the QHCP is warranted. When creating a query, it is important that all pertinent data and treatment directed toward the condition be identified within the context of the query. The introduction to appendix C provides straightforward guidance for writing an effective query.

Appendix D is a list of terms and their commonly used abbreviations. See the boxed text below for more guidance in using this appendix.

The following two pieces of information are also important for guiding the coder. First, the coder must follow the Uniform Hospital Discharge Data Set guidelines when deciding to code an "other additional diagnosis," commonly known as a secondary diagnosis. The definition of a secondary diagnosis is interpreted as additional conditions that affect patient care in terms of requiring:

- clinical evaluation,
- therapeutic treatment,
- diagnostic procedures,
- extended length of hospital stay, or
- increasing nursing care and/or monitoring.

Second, the appropriate use of health record documentation from non-physician health care providers is acceptable for serving as a basis for code assignments, as long as the non-physician providers are considered legally accountable for establishing a diagnosis within the regulations governing the provider and the facility. Each diagnosis assignment in this workbook reflects the scope of practice for the state in which the health record was created.

> *More on Appendix D . . .* Abbreviations of common terms are used throughout the workbook and answer key. For example, the initialism "QHCP" represents "qualified health care provider." Please refer to the list of abbreviations in appendix D for help in interpreting any of the common abbreviations used in the workbook and answer key. The list is in alphabetical order by abbreviation.

# ICD-9-CM and POA Coding Mentor

# Diseases and Disorders
# of the Nervous System

## BASIC HEALTH RECORD

At times, a patient will present with symptoms of slurred speech, dysphasia, weakness of the extremities, and facial droop. These are good clinical indicators for the diagnosis of a CVA, also commonly known as a stroke.

When documentation of a CVA is found in the patient's health record, it will be helpful for the coder to refer to the CVA sections in appendixes A and B for assistance in applying the specific codes required for this diagnosis. Also contained in these appendixes are the clinical indicators and description of a CVA.

When coding a record with this diagnosis, it is prudent to review the CAT scan, MRI, ECG (also called EKG), ultrasounds, and laboratory data to gain insight into the cause of the CVA and to determine whether any indicators for other diagnoses are relevant to the patient.

For coding a diagnosis of CVA, it is important to determine whether the condition is ischemic, embolic, or hemorrhagic. If the CVA is hemorrhagic, further clarification is needed to discover whether it was traumatic or non-traumatic.

Make sure to review the record closely for treatment of the CVA with tPA or any invasive procedures. In addition, knowing the location of the stroke and any lasting deficits that result is imperative.

When a diagnosis of respiratory insufficiency is noted in the patient's health record, it is important for the coder to recognize that the acuity of the condition needs to be documented by the QHCP in order to apply an accurate code. The coder cannot assume the acuity of the condition or diagnosis and, in some instances, will have to query the QHCP.

Based on the provided inpatient setting documentation, please assign the following:

- MS-DRG assignment
- ICD-9-CM diagnosis and procedure codes (FY2010)
- POA indicators

| MS-DRG Assignment |
| --- |
| |

| ICD-9-CM Diagnosis Codes | ICD-9-CM Diagnosis Description | POA | Coding Clinic Reference/Reason |
| --- | --- | --- | --- |
| | | | |
| | | | |
| | | | |
| | | | |
| | | | |
| | | | |
| | | | |
| | | | |
| | | | |
| | | | |
| | | | |
| | | | |
| | | | |
| | | | |
| | | | |

| ICD-9-CM Procedure Codes | ICD-9-CM Procedure Description |
|---|---|
|  |  |
|  |  |
|  |  |
|  |  |
|  |  |

| Query for QHCP |
|---|
|  |

# INTERMEDIATE HEALTH RECORD

When patients present to the hospital with a symptom that is caused by an underlying disease process, determining which studies are obtained by the coder depends on the symptom and can include laboratory data; x-rays; MRI results; a CAT scan; ultrasounds; or, at times, invasive tests, all of which may help the QHCP to determine a final diagnosis.

Review the entire health record for documentation or indications of secondary diagnoses that will assist in accurately reflecting the entire clinical scenario. Refer to ICD-9-CM coding guidelines for the appropriateness of applying V codes and the circumstances of their use.

Once the final diagnosis—in this case, seizure—is established, the coder must determine if the episode was a single occurrence or if the seizure was described as recurrent or as a seizure disorder. This determination will allow him or her to apply the most correct code. Coding guidelines address this topic.

When diagnoses are provided within reports, the QHCP is responsible for including those findings as diagnoses within the progress notes when appropriate. If the findings are not incorporated into the notes by the QHCP, the coder should query to determine if the findings constitute a diagnosis applicable to the patient and if they are clinically significant. For guidance in writing an appropriate query, refer to the examples in appendix C.

Based on the provided inpatient setting documentation, please assign the following:

- MS-DRG assignment
- ICD-9-CM diagnosis and procedure codes (FY2010)
- POA indicators

**MS-DRG Assignment**

| ICD-9-CM Diagnosis Codes | ICD-9-CM Diagnosis Description | POA | Coding Clinic Reference/Reason |
|---|---|---|---|
|  |  |  |  |
|  |  |  |  |
|  |  |  |  |
|  |  |  |  |
|  |  |  |  |
|  |  |  |  |
|  |  |  |  |
|  |  |  |  |
|  |  |  |  |
|  |  |  |  |
|  |  |  |  |
|  |  |  |  |
|  |  |  |  |
|  |  |  |  |

| ICD-9-CM Procedure Codes | ICD-9-CM Procedure Description |
|---|---|
|  |  |
|  |  |
|  |  |
|  |  |
|  |  |

| Query for QHCP |
|---|
|  |

## ADVANCED HEALTH RECORD

Injuries to the head and brain can produce effects that may require treatment long after the initial injury has occurred. When reviewing records of patients with brain injuries or brain conditions, it is imperative to determine the final diagnosis to assign the most accurate codes.

Multiple diagnosis codes may be assigned to describe the patient's condition in its entirety, and multiple procedure codes may be assigned to capture each procedure performed. Be attentive when abnormal findings are given, such as fever, leukocytosis, and elevated glucose measurements, as these may require additional tests or examinations by the QHCP to rule out potential complications or further diagnoses for the patient's hospitalization.

If, after the coder has thoroughly studied the record, no additional specified diagnoses are determined, it is appropriate to code the abnormal findings to justify length of stay, additional studies, or treatment directed toward an abnormal finding.

Based on the provided inpatient setting documentation, please assign the following:

* MS-DRG assignment
* ICD-9-CM diagnosis and procedure codes (FY2010)
* POA indicators

| | MS-DRG Assignment | | |
|---|---|---|---|

| ICD-9-CM Diagnosis Codes | ICD-9-CM Diagnosis Description | POA | Coding Clinic Reference/Reason |
|---|---|---|---|
| | | | |
| | | | |
| | | | |
| | | | |
| | | | |
| | | | |
| | | | |
| | | | |
| | | | |
| | | | |
| | | | |
| | | | |
| | | | |
| | | | |

| ICD-9-CM Procedure Codes | ICD-9-CM Procedure Description |
|---|---|
|  |  |
|  |  |
|  |  |
|  |  |
|  |  |

# CHAPTER 2

# Diseases and Disorders of the Eye

# BASIC HEALTH RECORD

Even though the eye is a relatively small organ, it has several separate components. Often, one or more of these components can become infected. It is important for the coder to determine all locations of the infection, including those surrounding the eye.

Several codes may be required to capture all infected sites. With any infection, careful study of the record will assist the coder in determining if the infection is localized or if indications are present of a systemic response to the localized infection.

Review of the sepsis sections in appendixes A and B will help the coder identify when a systemic response is present. If it appears that a systemic response is present but not documented as such in the patient's health record, the coder should consider querying the QHCP for clarification. The section of appendix C discussing a sepsis scenario will further assist the coder in generating such a query.

Per coding guidelines, when final coding of the record takes place, the systemic illness should appear first, followed by the localized infection(s).

All documented secondary diagnoses must meet one of the following five criteria for reporting additional diagnoses as outlined in the general coding guidelines on reporting additional diagnoses: (1) clinical evaluation, (2) therapeutic treatment, (3) diagnostic procedures, (4) extended length of hospital stay, and (5) increased nursing care and/or monitoring. These criteria should be considered for each secondary diagnosis. If none is met, the secondary diagnosis listed should be excluded from the coding.

Based on the provided inpatient setting documentation, please assign the following:

- MS-DRG assignment
- ICD-9-CM diagnosis codes (FY2010)
- POA indicators

| | MS-DRG Assignment | | |
|---|---|---|---|

| ICD-9-CM Diagnosis Codes | ICD-9-CM Diagnosis Description | POA | Coding Clinic Reference/Reason |
|---|---|---|---|
| | | | |
| | | | |
| | | | |
| | | | |
| | | | |
| | | | |
| | | | |
| | | | |
| | | | |
| | | | |

*ICD-9-CM and POA Coding Mentor,* edited by Patricia L. Bower-Jernigan, RHIA.

## INTERMEDIATE HEALTH RECORD

Retinal detachment is a serious condition that requires immediate medical attention. Patients may report sudden visual changes such as the appearance of flashes, objects floating in their visual field, shadows, and/or blurred vision.

With this condition, the retina detaches itself from the underlying tissue. Detachment is often associated with hemorrhage of the area. It is important for the coder to examine the patient's health record to identify a location, type, and/or cause of the detachment and hemorrhage(s). All locations of the hemorrhage(s) should be reported in the coding.

Blindness or visual impairment can be a lasting result of this condition. The ability to identify the level and type of impairment as well as which eye(s) is involved will aid the coder in achieving a greater specified code.

Furthermore, this acute visual loss can be a life-altering condition for a patient, and depression can result. Depression has several different causes and manifestations. The ability to capture the specifics of a diagnosis such as depression will lead to more detailed coding.

Mental disorders (such as dementia and depression) usually have a multitude of descriptors that, when identifiable in the record, can facilitate a more concise code assignment. When these diagnoses are only vaguely described in the patient's record, the coder must determine if a query is needed. Appendix C is a useful tool to assist in creating a query.

Diagnoses and their prophylactic (preventive) treatment may be documented in the record. These are not considered actual diagnoses, however, and should not be considered for coding. The QHCP is simply stating in the record that a treatment is provided to protect the patient from occurrence of these diagnoses.

Based on the provided inpatient setting documentation, please assign the following:

- MS-DRG assignment
- ICD-9-CM diagnosis and procedure codes (FY2010)
- POA indicators

| | MS-DRG Assignment | | |
|---|---|---|---|

| ICD-9-CM Diagnosis Codes | ICD-9-CM Diagnosis Description | POA | Coding Clinic Reference/Reason |
|---|---|---|---|
| | | | |
| | | | |
| | | | |
| | | | |
| | | | |
| | | | |
| | | | |
| | | | |
| | | | |
| | | | |
| | | | |
| | | | |
| | | | |

| ICD-9-CM Procedure Codes | ICD-9-CM Procedure Description |
|---|---|
|  |  |
|  |  |
|  |  |
|  |  |
|  |  |

| Query for QHCP |
|---|
|  |

| Query for QHCP |
|---|
|  |

# ADVANCED HEALTH RECORD

When reviewing a trauma record, it is imperative that the coder identify those areas of the body that have been affected. Understanding that deeper and surrounding areas of a traumatic wound can also be involved will assist the coder in identifying which codes should be applied.

When injury is sustained to the eye, the coder should look for involvement of all components of the eye itself, including the surrounding tissue and bone. If the wound is deep, close attention should be paid to any testing and monitoring for injury to the brain.

Test results of CAT scans and MRIs should be reviewed to see if diagnoses appear within these reports but are not identified by the QHCP in his or her documentation. These may require further clarification from the QHCP. Tests of this type should also be reported through the codes.

Mental status or behavioral changes, complaints of persistent headaches, sudden nausea and vomiting, changes in physical ability (such as speech impairment or weakness of a body part), and seizures are some physical clues of a deeper trauma that may involve the brain.

Infections can also result from trauma. The ability to capture all the diagnoses that are involved with the trauma injury will result in a complete depiction of the injury to the patient through the coding report. With any trauma, E codes should be applied to capture the type of injury and its location.

Insult to body structures often will need repair through surgical intervention. These interventions may occur at any time during the hospital stay. Close review of all documentation of procedures performed both inside and outside the operating room will allow the coder to capture all procedures performed.

Based on the provided inpatient setting documentation, please assign the following:

- MS-DRG assignment
- ICD-9-CM diagnosis and procedure codes (FY2010)
- POA indicators

| MS-DRG Assignment |
|---|
| |

| ICD-9-CM Diagnosis Codes | ICD-9-CM Diagnosis Description | POA | Coding Clinic Reference/Reason |
|---|---|---|---|
| | | | |
| | | | |
| | | | |
| | | | |
| | | | |
| | | | |
| | | | |
| | | | |
| | | | |
| | | | |

| ICD-9-CM Procedure Codes | ICD-9-CM Procedure Description |
|---|---|
| | |
| | |
| | |
| | |
| | |

# CHAPTER 3

# Diseases and Disorders of the Ear, Nose, Mouth and Throat

## BASIC HEALTH RECORD

Upon the patient's admission to the hospital, in this case due to dizziness, it is the responsibility of the QHCP to conduct a thorough examination of the patient and his or her medical history, including a review of the patient's complaints, medical and surgical history, and any other relevant findings that may provide clues as to the underlying cause of the presenting symptom.

After making the assessment, the QHCP typically orders diagnostic testing to aid in obtaining a final diagnosis. An MRI, laboratory work, and angiography may be ordered to rule out brain tumors, CVAs, and other anomalies of the brain or nervous system with a symptom such as dizziness. When a patient is feeling off balance or experiencing dizziness or a spinning sensation, for example, a diagnosis of a labyrinthine disorder or dysfunction is at times uncovered after other diagnoses are ruled out.

Any time a trauma to the head has occurred, disruption of the inner ear mechanisms is possible, but this disruption can be present when no inciting event, such as head trauma, has occurred. Inner ear disruption not caused by head trauma is considered idiopathic. Refer to appendix A for common diagnoses that often present with the symptom of dizziness.

Based on the provided inpatient setting documentation, please assign the following:

* MS-DRG assignment
* ICD-9-CM diagnosis and procedure codes (FY2010)
* POA indicators

| MS-DRG Assignment |
|---|
|  |

| ICD-9-CM Diagnosis Codes | ICD-9-CM Diagnosis Description | POA | Coding Clinic Reference/Reason |
|---|---|---|---|
|  |  |  |  |
|  |  |  |  |
|  |  |  |  |
|  |  |  |  |
|  |  |  |  |

| ICD-9-CM Procedure Codes | ICD-9-CM Procedure Description |
|---|---|
|  |  |
|  |  |
|  |  |
|  |  |
|  |  |

## INTERMEDIATE HEALTH RECORD

Dizziness and syncope can be common complaints of a patient presenting for care to the hospital. A battery of tests is often required to reveal the underlying cause or causes of these symptoms. The QHCP will often need to direct treatment at suspected, possible, or probable diagnoses, as the precipitating cause(s) may be elusive or unable to be reproduced during the hospitalization. For information on applying codes for diagnoses that are documented as being suspected, possible, or probable, refer to coding guidelines.

Peripheral vertigo is described as a feeling of spinning and occurs with movement of the head. It frequently causes nausea and vomiting. The patient may have the sensation of falling, moving, or spinning. Peripheral vertigo is frequently caused by problems within the inner ear.

Syncope and dizziness can have multiple causes; refer to the "Dizziness" workflow process tool in appendix A.

Occasions arise when writing a query to the QHCP would be helpful in obtaining further specificity of a diagnosis in terms of acuity, type, location, or stage. For guidelines in writing an appropriate query, refer to appendix C.

Based on the provided inpatient setting documentation, please assign the following:

- MS-DRG assignment
- ICD-9-CM diagnosis and procedure codes (FY2010)
- POA indicators

| | MS-DRG Assignment | | |
|---|---|---|---|
| | | | |

| ICD-9-CM Diagnosis Codes | ICD-9-CM Diagnosis Description | POA | Coding Clinic Reference/Reason |
|---|---|---|---|
| | | | |
| | | | |
| | | | |
| | | | |
| | | | |
| | | | |
| | | | |
| | | | |
| | | | |
| | | | |
| | | | |
| | | | |
| | | | |

*(Continued on next page)*

| ICD-9-CM Diagnosis Codes | ICD-9-CM Diagnosis Description | POA | Coding Clinic Reference/Reason |
|---|---|---|---|
|  |  |  |  |
|  |  |  |  |
|  |  |  |  |
|  |  |  |  |
|  |  |  |  |
|  |  |  |  |

| ICD-9-CM Procedure Codes | ICD-9-CM Procedure Description |
|---|---|
|  |  |
|  |  |
|  |  |
|  |  |
|  |  |

| Query for QHCP |
|---|
|  |

# ADVANCED HEALTH RECORD

In the event that a patient presents for elective surgery, it is imperative that the coder review the entire record for documentation of diagnoses pertaining to all body systems. In this case, neoplasms that are found in the mouth, throat, nose, or ear can affect numerous body systems and, depending on their location, can cause major changes in the patient's ability to take nourishment, breathe, and speak.

When the patient is scheduled to undergo surgery for a mass or tumor that has not yet been identified, it is critical for the QHCP to document the pathological identification of primary and metastatic or invasive sites in the progress notes or discharge summary when they become available. The coder cannot code results from the pathology reports until the QHCP has attested to them through documentation.

It is appropriate for the coder to query the QHCP in cases in which the pathology is not identified within the notes in order to obtain specified and accurate diagnoses. The coder must have an understanding of the coding guidelines to be able to apply the most accurate diagnoses and procedure codes to a coding abstract.

When conflicting information is documented within the patient's health record, a query is appropriate. See appendix C for guidelines in writing queries.

Based on the provided inpatient setting documentation, please assign the following:

- MS-DRG assignment
- ICD-9-CM diagnosis and procedure codes (FY2010)
- POA indicators

| MS-DRG Assignment |
|---|
| |

| ICD-9-CM Diagnosis Codes | ICD-9-CM Diagnosis Description | POA | Coding Clinic Reference/Reason |
|---|---|---|---|
| | | | |
| | | | |
| | | | |
| | | | |
| | | | |
| | | | |
| | | | |
| | | | |
| | | | |
| | | | |

| ICD-9-CM Procedure Codes | ICD-9-CM Procedure Description |
|---|---|
|  |  |
|  |  |
|  |  |
|  |  |
|  |  |
|  |  |
|  |  |
|  |  |
|  |  |
|  |  |

| Query for QHCP |
|---|
|  |

# Diseases and Disorders
# of the Respiratory System

## BASIC HEALTH RECORD

Many conditions can affect a patient's respiratory status. When a patient presents with symptoms such as shortness of breath, tachypnea, and hypoxia, the QHCP may list several possible diagnoses in the patient's health record that will require testing and monitoring in order to determine the final diagnosis or diagnoses.

It is not uncommon for more than one diagnosis to be identified through this process as the cause of the presenting symptoms. Careful review of the patient's record will assist the coder in identifying the most appropriate principal diagnoses.

When all the listed diagnoses meet the criteria for principal diagnosis, the coder may choose which diagnosis will be listed as principal. Many times, diagnoses are still under evaluation and treatment, and the coder cannot determine if they have been confirmed by the QHCP. When the QHCP notes these diagnoses as possible, probable, or suspected, it is appropriate to assign codes for these diagnoses. This rule applies to neoplasm and the metastatic sites as well. Coding guidelines and *Coding Clinic* are available for review on this subject.

The coder should always remember to assess the documentation for respiratory impairments, such as failure or distress, in patients with those symptoms identified in this health record. This assessment will help the coder determine if further clarification from the QHCP is required for possible additional diagnoses. Refer to appendixes A, B, and C for assessment and querying guidelines on acute and chronic respiratory failure.

Also available to coders for reference are specific guidelines on what codes to apply for patients whose diagnoses are closely related, such as COPD and asthma. These diagnoses will not be coded separately, as the chronic disease process will incorporate the asthma into a single code.

When diagnoses such as CHF, anemia, and pneumonia are documented without further descriptions of acuity, type, or cause, it is important for the coder to review test results and treatment plans to determine if the QHCP may be able to clarify a more specific diagnosis.

When a coder suspects that a more specific diagnosis could be documented or if it is too difficult to determine whether a description could be further clarified, it is appropriate for him or her to query the QHCP. Appendixes A, B, and C will be useful in these situations.

Initial diagnoses may appear in the patient's health record that subsequent testing eliminated. In such a case, a code should not be applied for that initial diagnosis.

Based on the provided inpatient setting documentation, please assign the following:

- MS-DRG assignment
- ICD-9-CM diagnosis and procedure codes (FY2010)
- POA indicators

| MS-DRG Assignment |
| --- |
|  |

| ICD-9-CM Diagnosis Codes | ICD-9-CM Diagnosis Description | POA | Coding Clinic Reference/Reason |
| --- | --- | --- | --- |
|  |  |  |  |
|  |  |  |  |
|  |  |  |  |
|  |  |  |  |
|  |  |  |  |
|  |  |  |  |
|  |  |  |  |
|  |  |  |  |
|  |  |  |  |
|  |  |  |  |
|  |  |  |  |
|  |  |  |  |
|  |  |  |  |
|  |  |  |  |

| ICD-9-CM Procedure Codes | ICD-9-CM Procedure Description |
|---|---|
| | |
| | |
| | |
| | |
| | |

## INTERMEDIATE HEALTH RECORD

Patients with chronic, debilitating diagnoses such as COPD, cancers, and heart disease with heart failure are often subject to repeat admissions to the hospital setting. The presence of acute conditions coupled with chronic debilitating diagnoses often leads to a complication such as pneumonia. This condition can result from limited physical activity and airway exchange in addition to exposure to a multitude of bacteria and viruses in a health care environment. Review of the pneumonia and acute respiratory failure sections in appendixes A and B will guide the coder in determining if a query for any clarification on these diagnoses is needed.

With patients who have chronic diagnoses that impair the respiratory function, review of the treatment plan for conditions such as oxygen dependency can be beneficial in determining additional codes.

Because each diagnosis's treatment plan will affect another diagnosis, it can be difficult to control all these diagnoses in a single patient record. Renal function is often affected in patients with co-morbidities. For example, fluid may be administered for one diagnosis, but the additional fluid may result in fluid overload or exacerbation of pre-existing heart failure.

When chronic kidney disease already exists, it is not uncommon for acute renal failure to occur. Many QHCPs refer to this condition by interchangeable terms such as *acute renal failure*, *acute renal insufficiency*, and *acute kidney injury*. *Coding Clinic* has recently advised that the term *acute kidney injury* is acceptable and equal to *acute renal failure* in meaning. However, the diagnosis of acute renal insufficiency is not to be considered interchangeable with that of acute renal failure. It is important for the coder to determine which diagnosis is noted most frequently and whether acute renal failure truly exists based on laboratory results and treatment surrounding it. A query to the QHCP is appropriate when this determination cannot be made.

Furthermore, chronic kidney disease requires additional description by its stage for the most accurate code to be applied. The sections on renal failure in appendix A will be of use to the coder in this scenario.

Based on the provided inpatient setting documentation, please assign the following:

- MS-DRG assignment
- ICD-9-CM diagnosis and procedure codes (FY2010)
- POA indicators

| MS-DRG Assignment | | | |
|---|---|---|---|

| ICD-9-CM Diagnosis Codes | ICD-9-CM Diagnosis Description | POA | Coding Clinic Reference/Reason |
|---|---|---|---|
| | | | |
| | | | |
| | | | |
| | | | |
| | | | |
| | | | |
| | | | |
| | | | |
| | | | |
| | | | |
| | | | |
| | | | |
| | | | |

*(Continued on next page)*

Diseases and Disorders of the Respiratory System

| ICD-9-CM Diagnosis Codes | ICD-9-CM Diagnosis Description | POA | Coding Clinic Reference/Reason |
|---|---|---|---|
|  |  |  |  |
|  |  |  |  |
|  |  |  |  |
|  |  |  |  |
|  |  |  |  |
|  |  |  |  |
|  |  |  |  |
|  |  |  |  |
|  |  |  |  |
|  |  |  |  |
|  |  |  |  |
|  |  |  |  |
|  |  |  |  |
|  |  |  |  |
|  |  |  |  |

*ICD-9-CM and POA Coding Mentor,* edited by Patricia L. Bower-Jernigan, RHIA.
Copyright ©2010 Health Forum, Inc., an American Hospital Association company. All rights reserved.

| ICD-9-CM Procedure Codes | ICD-9-CM Procedure Description |
|---|---|
|  |  |
|  |  |
|  |  |
|  |  |
|  |  |

| Query for QHCP |
|---|
|  |

# ADVANCED HEALTH RECORD

When a patient is admitted following or currently in a cardiac or respiratory arrest, it is important to identify the cause of the arrest to help determine the principal diagnosis. If the cause is determined, the arrest should not be sequenced as the principal diagnosis in the coding abstract. Specific coding guidelines state that the underlying cause of the arrest should be sequenced first. Only in situations where the cause is not determined should the arrest be coded as principal.

Acute respiratory failure is a life-threatening condition that requires a vast amount of resources to treat. When artificial ventilation is one of the treatments provided, it is imperative for the coder to examine the duration of its use. The determination of less than or greater than ninety-six hours of artificial ventilation is required for proper coding assignment. Often, nursing and respiratory care notes or flow sheets can be helpful in determining duration of artificial ventilation hours if the QHCP's notes are not clear on this time frame. The sections on acute respiratory failure in appendixes A and B will serve as a guide for coding related to patients with acute respiratory failure.

Arrests and failures often affect other body systems as well. Thus, careful review of the record allows the coder to capture the impact of the arrest and failure(s) through the codes assigned.

Mental impairment often follows an arrest because of the depletion of oxygen to the brain. Review of the record for conditions such as specified types of encephalopathy, anoxic brain damage, or coma is imperative. It is common for a patient with impaired mental status in addition to respiratory compromise to have frank or silent aspiration. This aspiration of a patient's own saliva or secretions may result in aspiration pneumonia. Review of the sections on pneumonia in appendixes A and B will help guide the coder in determining whether a query is required for further clarification of a particular type or cause of a documented pneumonia.

Identifying the specific types and causes of these diagnoses as well as other additional diagnoses will allow for a precise coding abstract.

Based on the provided inpatient setting documentation, please assign the following:

- MS-DRG assignment
- ICD-9-CM diagnosis and procedure codes (FY2010)
- POA indicators

| MS-DRG Assignment |
|---|
| |

| ICD-9-CM Diagnosis Codes | ICD-9-CM Diagnosis Description | POA | Coding Clinic Reference/Reason |
|---|---|---|---|
| | | | |
| | | | |
| | | | |
| | | | |
| | | | |
| | | | |
| | | | |
| | | | |
| | | | |
| | | | |
| | | | |
| | | | |
| | | | |
| | | | |

| ICD-9-CM Procedure Codes | ICD-9-CM Procedure Description |
|---|---|
| | |
| | |
| | |
| | |
| | |
| | |
| | |
| | |
| | |
| | |

# CHAPTER 5

# Diseases and Disorders of the Circulatory System

## BASIC HEALTH RECORD

When a patient is admitted with two potential principal diagnoses, identifying the principal diagnosis requires attention to the evaluation, monitoring, and treatment plan documented in the patient's health record. If both diagnoses are treated equally—that is, with the same evaluation process, monitoring, and treatment plan—the coder can make the choice between the two diagnoses for assignment of principal diagnosis as long as no specified guideline exists stating otherwise. Review of coding guidelines and *Coding Clinic* will help the coder identify when this rule applies.

When coding records with heart failure, it is important to remember that the acuity of heart failure can be affected by several driving forces. Changes in heart rate or type of rhythm, changes in existing treatment plan, and heart structure abnormalities are some of the more influential factors that cause an increase in acuity or are attributed to the chronic state of the disease.

Evaluation through a variety of tests and/or monitoring often takes place during the hospitalization. When the QHCP establishes the cause of the acute or chronic heart failure, the coder can then determine the proper code(s) to capture the greatest specificity.

It is not uncommon for heart failure patients to have more than one cause for their condition, especially in relationship to the acuity. Acute heart failure occurrences may result because of a rapid change in the patient's existing treatment plan; they may develop when he or she is not compliant with treatment or when a new treatment is given to him or her, such as increase in fluid intake. This may be identified in the QHCP's documentation in cases of impaired kidney function. Rapid change in heart rate or rhythm type as well as progressive or acute changes in heart structure can also result in acute heart failure.

Chronic heart failure, on the other hand, is more often influenced by structural changes such as impaired diastolic or systolic ventricular function and prolonged valvular disease. If a coder identifies the possibility that not all causes for either the acute or chronic heart failure are described in the record, careful examination of test results, such as ECGs, are key in determining if a query should be sent to the QHCP for further clarification. The sections on heart failure in appendixes B and C will serve as useful tools.

Based on the provided inpatient setting documentation, please assign the following:

- MS-DRG assignment
- ICD-9-CM diagnosis and procedure codes (FY2010)
- POA indicators

| MS-DRG Assignment |
|---|
| |

| ICD-9-CM Diagnosis Codes | ICD-9-CM Diagnosis Description | POA | Coding Clinic Reference/Reason |
|---|---|---|---|
| | | | |
| | | | |
| | | | |
| | | | |
| | | | |
| | | | |
| | | | |
| | | | |
| | | | |
| | | | |

| ICD-9-CM Procedure Codes | ICD-9-CM Procedure Description |
|---|---|
|  |  |
|  |  |
|  |  |
|  |  |
|  |  |

| Query for QHCP |
|---|
|  |

## INTERMEDIATE HEALTH RECORD

Percutaneous transluminal coronary interventions are widely used in treatment of CAD. They are less invasive than open heart surgery and are effective ways to clear or reduce blockage of the coronary arteries.

When reviewing a chart showing that a percutaneous transluminal coronary intervention took place, it is best to review the actual procedure note or log. The type of procedure, number of vessels, and type of devices deployed need to be identified in order to assign the proper procedure codes.

When stents are used in the intervention, it is imperative that the coder identify whether the stent is drug eluting or bare metal. Progress notes may identify a brand name for the stent(s), but the QHCP should identify the stent type as either drug eluting or bare metal before the coder assigns the proper code(s). Often, more than one type of stent is deployed during a procedure, depending on the vessel, location of the stenosis within the vessel, degree of stenosis, and patient's overall health status and treatment regimen.

The number of deployed stents is not always easy to identify in progress notes, but review of the procedure note or log should help with this determination. Assignment by DRG is dependent on the type of stent deployed as well as the number of stents deployed.

All secondary diagnoses should also be identified, by stage or degree when applicable, to achieve the most complete description of causal relationship. When renal impairment is determined by the QHCP to be linked to diagnoses such as hypertension or diabetes, diligent assignment of codes is required. When a QHCP documents more than one stage, it is at the coder's discretion to assign one of the documented stages. The coder should consider a query if determination of which stage to assign is uncertain.

Based on the provided inpatient setting documentation, please assign the following:

* MS-DRG assignment
* ICD-9-CM diagnosis and procedure codes (FY2010)
* POA indicators

| MS-DRG Assignment |
|---|
|  |

| ICD-9-CM Diagnosis Codes | ICD-9-CM Diagnosis Description | POA | Coding Clinic Reference/Reason |
|---|---|---|---|
|  |  |  |  |
|  |  |  |  |
|  |  |  |  |
|  |  |  |  |
|  |  |  |  |
|  |  |  |  |
|  |  |  |  |
|  |  |  |  |
|  |  |  |  |
|  |  |  |  |
|  |  |  |  |
|  |  |  |  |
|  |  |  |  |
|  |  |  |  |
|  |  |  |  |

| ICD-9-CM Procedure Codes | ICD-9-CM Procedure Description |
|---|---|
| | |
| | |
| | |
| | |
| | |
| | |
| | |
| | |
| | |
| | |

## ADVANCED HEALTH RECORD

Patients who present to the hospital with AMI often are evaluated with a battery of tests. The AMI section of appendix B is a useful tool for coders in helping understand this condition.

Angiograms are frequently performed to assess the cause of the AMI. In many situations, the treatment plan will depend on the results of the angiogram. Interventions such as PTCA with or without stent placement can be a first choice of treatment.

However, the patient may not be a suitable candidate for this form of treatment, so a CABG may be considered the best intervention. When the coronary arteries are severely compromised, an intra-aortic balloon pump may be placed to increase the blood flow to the arteries before and after the bypass is performed. Attention should be given to the number of vessels grafted when a bypass is performed.

Patients with such complex cases can often experience complications following surgery. A thorough review of all secondary diagnoses should be conducted to help the coder determine if each diagnosis is described by its acuity, stage, degree, type, and cause. The patient's chronic conditions also must be reviewed to determine if they are being addressed with a current treatment plan. The coder should assess each secondary diagnosis to determine if it meets the criteria per coding guidelines. Refer to the "How to Use This Workbook" section for the five criteria for secondary diagnoses.

Based on the provided inpatient setting documentation, please assign the following:

- MS-DRG assignment
- ICD-9-CM diagnosis and procedure codes (FY2010)
- POA indicators

| | MS-DRG Assignment | | |
|---|---|---|---|
| | | | |

| ICD-9-CM Diagnosis Codes | ICD-9-CM Diagnosis Description | POA | Coding Clinic Reference/Reason |
|---|---|---|---|
| | | | |
| | | | |
| | | | |
| | | | |
| | | | |
| | | | |
| | | | |
| | | | |
| | | | |
| | | | |
| | | | |
| | | | |
| | | | |
| | | | |

*(Continued on next page)*

*ICD-9-CM and POA Coding Mentor,* edited by Patricia L. Bower-Jernigan, RHIA.

| ICD-9-CM Diagnosis Codes | ICD-9-CM Diagnosis Description | POA | Coding Clinic Reference/Reason |
|---|---|---|---|
| | | | |
| | | | |
| | | | |
| | | | |
| | | | |
| | | | |
| | | | |
| | | | |
| | | | |
| | | | |
| | | | |
| | | | |
| | | | |
| | | | |
| | | | |

| ICD-9-CM Procedure Codes | ICD-9-CM Procedure Description |
|---|---|
|  |  |
|  |  |
|  |  |
|  |  |
|  |  |
|  |  |
|  |  |
|  |  |
|  |  |
|  |  |
|  |  |
|  |  |
|  |  |
|  |  |

# Diseases and Disorders of the Digestive System

## BASIC HEALTH RECORD

When patients present to the hospital with abdominal pain coupled with bloating and decreasing regularity or lack of bowel movements, these symptoms are strongly suggestive of a bowel obstruction.

Some patients experience repeated bowel obstructions due to underlying medical conditions such as adhesions, cystic fibrosis, or carcinoma. Cystic fibrosis is a condition in which the patient has very sticky and thick mucous that often complicates other body systems, including the respiratory and gastrointestinal tracts.

Be mindful of secondary findings in patients with bowel obstructions, such as dehydration, electrolyte abnormalities, and nausea and vomiting. Specific coding guidelines direct the coder to proper sequencing when the patient has a diagnosis of cystic fibrosis. If the coder needs additional details in order to assign a more specified code, a query should be written. Refer to appendix C for direction in writing queries.

Based on the provided inpatient setting documentation, please assign the following:

- MS-DRG assignment
- ICD-9-CM diagnosis and procedure codes (FY2010)
- POA indicators

| MS-DRG Assignment |
| --- |
|  |

| ICD-9-CM Diagnosis Codes | ICD-9-CM Diagnosis Description | POA | Coding Clinic Reference/Reason |
| --- | --- | --- | --- |
|  |  |  |  |
|  |  |  |  |
|  |  |  |  |
|  |  |  |  |
|  |  |  |  |

| ICD-9-CM Procedure Codes | ICD-9-CM Procedure Description |
| --- | --- |
|  |  |
|  |  |
|  |  |
|  |  |
|  |  |

**Query for QHCP**

## INTERMEDIATE HEALTH RECORD

Clinical indicators for a gastrointestinal hemorrhage include bloody or dark stools, hypotension, a drop in hemoglobin, light-headedness, and sometimes a history of a gastrointestinal hemorrhage.

After results of studies have been obtained, the QHCP can often identify the underlying cause and the site of the bleeding. He or she must link the findings in the studies to the gastrointestinal hemorrhage; the coder cannot assume the linkage. Coding guidelines advise on proper selection of code(s) in the event that a site appears to be healed at the time of endoscopy but the QHCP documents a hemorrhage.

It is necessary to review the entire health record for secondary diagnoses commonly associated with this diagnosis, such as acute blood-loss anemia, chronic blood-loss anemia, hypotension, dehydration, and shock (hemorrhagic or hypovolemic).

At times, a patient will be admitted to the hospital under treatment for a problem that was diagnosed prior to the current encounter. If the patient is still under treatment for that condition, the coder should code it as current. If clinical indicators are present for an additional diagnosis but one is not documented, it is appropriate for the coder to query the QHCP.

Based on the provided inpatient setting documentation, please assign the following:

- MS-DRG assignment
- ICD-9-CM diagnosis and procedure codes (FY2010)
- POA indicators

CHAPTER 6

| | MS-DRG Assignment | | |
|---|---|---|---|

| ICD-9-CM Diagnosis Codes | ICD-9-CM Diagnosis Description | POA | Coding Clinic Reference/Reason |
|---|---|---|---|
| | | | |
| | | | |
| | | | |
| | | | |
| | | | |
| | | | |
| | | | |
| | | | |
| | | | |
| | | | |
| | | | |
| | | | |
| | | | |
| | | | |

*ICD-9-CM and POA Coding Mentor,* edited by Patricia L. Bower-Jernigan, RHIA.

| ICD-9-CM Procedure Codes | ICD-9-CM Procedure Description |
|---|---|
|  |  |
|  |  |
|  |  |
|  |  |
|  |  |

## ADVANCED HEALTH RECORD

Masses within the gastrointestinal tract are often removed and tested to define the pathology (primary and secondary sites) and to prevent complications. Masses can be identified as benign, malignant, or unspecified. After studies are conducted, it is the responsibility of the QHCP to document the pathological findings within the progress notes or discharge summary.

Reviewing the entire health record will assist the coder in assigning codes for all secondary diagnoses relevant to the patient. Refer to the "How to Use This Workbook" section for the five criteria for secondary diagnoses. When any discrepancy arises within the documentation regarding a diagnosis or a procedure, and after review the coder is unable to determine the record's accuracy, the coder is obligated to query the QHCP for the proper documentation.

Based on the provided inpatient setting documentation, please assign the following:

- MS-DRG assignment
- ICD-9-CM diagnosis and procedure codes (FY2010)
- POA indicators

| MS-DRG Assignment |
| --- |
|  |

| ICD-9-CM Diagnosis Codes | ICD-9-CM Diagnosis Description | POA | Coding Clinic Reference/Reason |
| --- | --- | --- | --- |
|  |  |  |  |
|  |  |  |  |
|  |  |  |  |
|  |  |  |  |
|  |  |  |  |
|  |  |  |  |
|  |  |  |  |
|  |  |  |  |
|  |  |  |  |

| ICD-9-CM Procedure Codes | ICD-9-CM Procedure Description |
| --- | --- |
|  |  |
|  |  |
|  |  |
|  |  |
|  |  |

# Diseases and Disorders of the Hepatobiliary System and Pancreas

# BASIC HEALTH RECORD

Careful review of the clinical data, including laboratory results and CAT scans; the documentation within a patient's health record; and a physical description of the patient is key to determining the principal diagnosis that is best in keeping with the reason the patient presented for care.

Certain diagnoses are often associated with one another, and coding guidelines assist the coder in determining if sequencing rules need to be followd. By reviewing the documentation, including the operative note, a coder can at times obtain a diagnosis through coding logic. In other words, the description of the anatomy or of an organ from the QHCP can guide the coder to a specified code.

Based on the provided inpatient setting documentation, please assign the following:

- MS-DRG assignment
- ICD-9-CM diagnosis and procedure codes (FY2010)
- POA indicators

| MS-DRG Assignment |
|---|
| |

| ICD-9-CM Diagnosis Codes | ICD-9-CM Diagnosis Description | POA | Coding Clinic Reference/Reason |
|---|---|---|---|
| | | | |
| | | | |
| | | | |
| | | | |
| | | | |

| ICD-9-CM Procedure Codes | ICD-9-CM Procedure Description |
|---|---|
| | |
| | |
| | |
| | |
| | |

# INTERMEDIATE HEALTH RECORD

Often, a multitude of symptoms brings a patient to the hospital. Depending on these symptoms, testing is initiated to obtain a diagnosis. Once a diagnosis is determined, the coder needs to review the entire health record for secondary diagnoses that are commonly associated with it.

In the case of malignancies, secondary sites of cancer are often discovered or known, and the coder must be diligent in the review of the record to find notations of these.

Often, other body systems are affected in cancer cases, such as the skin and the gastrointestinal tract, including nutritional status and electrolyte imbalances, as is the patient's psychological state. The overall clinical picture of the patient should be discernible in the coding abstract.

Some procedures are performed to obtain a diagnosis, and some for the comfort of the patient. Not all procedures performed will affect the MS-DRG assignment.

Based on the provided inpatient setting documentation, please assign the following:

- MS-DRG assignment
- ICD-9-CM diagnosis and procedure codes (FY2010)
- POA indicators

| MS-DRG Assignment |
|---|
|  |

| ICD-9-CM Diagnosis Codes | ICD-9-CM Diagnosis Description | POA | Coding Clinic Reference/Reason |
|---|---|---|---|
|  |  |  |  |
|  |  |  |  |
|  |  |  |  |
|  |  |  |  |
|  |  |  |  |
|  |  |  |  |
|  |  |  |  |
|  |  |  |  |
|  |  |  |  |
|  |  |  |  |

| ICD-9-CM Procedure Codes | ICD-9-CM Procedure Description |
|---|---|
| | |
| | |
| | |
| | |
| | |
| | |
| | |
| | |
| | |
| | |

# ADVANCED HEALTH RECORD

Review of the entire health record is imperative in order to arrive at proper code assignment. When underlying conditions are described as the cause for an acute condition, it is the responsibility of the coder to determine if any coding guidelines are pertinent to the diagnoses for establishing the proper code assignment.

In some cases, the coding logic will dictate which diagnosis becomes the principal diagnosis. Intense review of the health record is necessary to reveal any secondary diagnoses. If clinical indicators are seen in physical descriptions of the patient, laboratory findings, x-rays, scans, or other studies that cause the coder to suspect additional diagnoses, it is appropriate for him or her to query the QHCP.

Note that patients who have chronic illnesses or conditions are more prone to alterations in skin integrity; changes in nutritional status; and, at times, difficulties with gastrointestinal disorders, to list a few secondary issues.

In this health record, a query has been written. Since the time it was prepared, more stringent guidelines have been established for the query process. For those guidelines, please see appendix C.

Based on the provided inpatient setting documentation, please assign the following:

- MS-DRG assignment
- ICD-9-CM diagnosis and procedure codes (FY2010)
- POA indicators

| | MS-DRG Assignment | | |
|---|---|---|---|

| ICD-9-CM Diagnosis Codes | ICD-9-CM Diagnosis Description | POA | Coding Clinic Reference/Reason |
|---|---|---|---|
| | | | |
| | | | |
| | | | |
| | | | |
| | | | |
| | | | |
| | | | |
| | | | |
| | | | |
| | | | |
| | | | |
| | | | |

*(Continued on next page)*

| ICD-9-CM Diagnosis Codes | ICD-9-CM Diagnosis Description | POA | Coding Clinic Reference/Reason |
|---|---|---|---|
| | | | |
| | | | |
| | | | |
| | | | |
| | | | |
| | | | |
| | | | |
| | | | |

| ICD-9-CM Procedure Codes | ICD-9-CM Procedure Description |
|---|---|
| | |
| | |
| | |
| | |
| | |

# CHAPTER 8

# Diseases and Disorders of the Musculoskeletal System and Connective Tissue

## BASIC HEALTH RECORD

When coding the record of a patient who is having back surgery, it is likely that the patient has had numerous treatment modalities prior to the decision to undergo surgery. It is helpful if the QHCP includes documentation of the type of disc disorder that is present. Common disc disorders involve degeneration, herniation, or infection.

It is necessary for the QHCP to specify any spinal cord damage as well as any underlying complications caused from the disc disorder, including bladder or bowel dysfunction, foot drop, parasthesia, or limitation of motion.

When reviewing the record, it is imperative for the coder to examine the operative note in its entirety to gain insight into the procedure(s) performed. Some spinal procedures when performed together are considered integral to one another and do not require separate codes. See coding guidelines for specific instructions.

If any additional secondary diagnoses are suspected that are not documented within the health record, the coder should query the QHCP for further clarification.

Based on the provided inpatient setting documentation, please assign the following:

- MS-DRG assignment
- ICD-9-CM diagnosis and procedure codes (FY2010)
- POA indicators

| MS-DRG Assignment |
| --- |
|  |

| ICD-9-CM Diagnosis Codes | ICD-9-CM Diagnosis Description | POA | Coding Clinic Reference/Reason |
| --- | --- | --- | --- |
|  |  |  |  |
|  |  |  |  |
|  |  |  |  |
|  |  |  |  |
|  |  |  |  |

| ICD-9-CM Procedure Codes | ICD-9-CM Procedure Description |
| --- | --- |
|  |  |
|  |  |
|  |  |
|  |  |
|  |  |

## INTERMEDIATE HEALTH RECORD

When patients present to the hospital for elective spinal fusion surgery, it is necessary for the coder to find the reason for the fusion (principal diagnosis) and determine the correct procedure codes. The reasons for spinal fusion can be related to injuries, deformities, instability of the spine, or pain.

Fusion of the spine is performed by inserting a bone graft between two or more vertebrae to eliminate the movement between them. Sometimes, a patient undergoes more than one spinal fusion procedure, and it may be the case that more than one surgeon performs the procedures. In such cases, both operative notes should be inspected for accurate code assignments.

Fusions may be anterior or posterior (or both), and they often involve insertion of hardware or devices. The coder needs to pay close attention to how many levels of the spine are fused.

Certain postoperative conditions are seen at times in relation to spinal fusion surgery, including a drop in hemoglobin, fever, arrhythmias, and electrolyte imbalances. After review of the health record, if the coder suspects that additional diagnoses could be appropriate for the patient that are not documented, a query should be written to the QHCP for clarification.

A query appears in this record. Since the time it was written, more stringent guidelines have been established for the query process. For assistance in those guidelines, refer to appendix C.

Based on the provided inpatient setting documentation, please assign the following:

- MS-DRG assignment
- ICD-9-CM diagnosis and procedure codes (FY2010)
- POA indicators

| MS-DRG Assignment |
| --- |
| |

| ICD-9-CM Diagnosis Codes | ICD-9-CM Diagnosis Description | POA | Coding Clinic Reference/Reason |
| --- | --- | --- | --- |
| | | | |
| | | | |
| | | | |
| | | | |
| | | | |

| ICD-9-CM Procedure Codes | ICD-9-CM Procedure Description |
| --- | --- |
| | |
| | |
| | |
| | |
| | |
| | |
| | |
| | |
| | |
| | |

## ADVANCED HEALTH RECORD

Fractures can be traumatic or non-traumatic. Non-traumatic fractures are also referred to as pathological, spontaneous, or insufficiency fractures. The diagnosis is uncovered by the use of x-rays and at times requires bone scans, MRIs, or CAT scans.

Fracture fixation is performed for both comfort and mobility. It is necessary for the coder to review the record in its entirety to apply accurate code assignments for the diagnoses and the procedures performed when applicable. The coder may need to query the QHCP at times to obtain a more specified diagnosis or further clarification of a diagnosis that is already documented. In this situation, there are secondary diagnoses that more specificity would reveal. Refer to appendix C for assistance in writing queries.

Based on the provided inpatient setting documentation, please assign the following:

- MS-DRG assignment
- ICD-9-CM diagnosis and procedure codes (FY2010)
- POA indicators

*ICD-9-CM and POA Coding Mentor,* edited by Patricia L. Bower-Jernigan, RHIA.

| MS-DRG Assignment |
| --- |
| |

| ICD-9-CM Diagnosis Codes | ICD-9-CM Diagnosis Description | POA | Coding Clinic Reference/Reason |
| --- | --- | --- | --- |
| | | | |
| | | | |
| | | | |
| | | | |
| | | | |
| | | | |
| | | | |
| | | | |
| | | | |
| | | | |
| | | | |
| | | | |

*(Continued on next page)*

| ICD-9-CM Diagnosis Codes | ICD-9-CM Diagnosis Description | POA | Coding Clinic Reference/Reason |
|---|---|---|---|
| | | | |
| | | | |
| | | | |
| | | | |
| | | | |
| | | | |
| | | | |
| | | | |

| ICD-9-CM Procedure Codes | ICD-9-CM Procedure Description |
|---|---|
| | |
| | |
| | |
| | |
| | |

**Query for QHCP**

**Query for QHCP**

# Diseases and Disorders of the Skin, Subcutaneous Tissue and Breast

## BASIC HEALTH RECORD

Inflammation of the skin and underlying tissue, referred to as cellulitis, is often described in the record as swelling, redness, increased warmth to the area, and associated pain. Also, fluid may be weeping from the site.

Skin ulceration is often associated with cellulitis. Careful review of the record will help in determining if the cellulitis is associated with a traumatic injury, a post-operative complication, or an ongoing chronic skin ulceration. If the organism(s) involved with the cellulitis is identified, additional codes for the organism(s) should be applied. All sites identified should be coded separately.

With all infections, the coder should review the patient's health record for SIRS. Sepsis is defined as SIRS with proven or suspected infection. When reviewing the record, look for the four indicators of SIRS identified in the section on sepsis in appendix B.

If two or more indicators are noted with a source of infection, the coder should look for documentation of sepsis. A query should be written asking the QHCP if SIRS and sepsis are additional diagnoses for the record when documentation of this is not found.

Review of the coding guidelines and *Coding Clinic* on sequencing systemic and localized infections should be performed to ensure proper sequencing of the principal diagnosis.

Electrolyte imbalances can often occur when the body is under stress due to infections or insults. Correct terminology related to the imbalance—not a notation of the abnormal finding by its value or by arrows signifying elevated or decreased levels—must appear within the QHCP's documentation before the diagnosis can be considered for coding. When a diagnosis is noted as "borderline," the coder should not consider this an actual diagnosis. A query should be generated requesting further clarification.

Based on the provided inpatient setting documentation, please assign the following:

- MS-DRG assignment
- ICD-9-CM diagnosis codes (FY2010)
- POA indicators

| MS-DRG Assignment |
| --- |
|  |

| ICD-9-CM Diagnosis Codes | ICD-9-CM Diagnosis Description | POA | Coding Clinic Reference/Reason |
| --- | --- | --- | --- |
|  |  |  |  |
|  |  |  |  |
|  |  |  |  |
|  |  |  |  |
|  |  |  |  |

| Query for QHCP |
| --- |
|  |

## INTERMEDIATE HEALTH RECORD

Infected skin ulcers are often accompanied by surrounding cellulitis. Attention should be paid to the treatment provided during the hospitalization to help establish the principal diagnosis.

When both infected skin ulcers and cellulitis meet the criteria for principal diagnosis, the coder may select which will be sequenced as principal. It is also important to review the record for systemic involvement. The sepsis sections in appendixes A and B should be reviewed when coding records pertaining to infection.

Identification of all sites, organisms, and causes of the ulcers and cellulitis is necessary. Site-specific codes are used for both skin ulcers and cellulitis. Careful review to capture all stated sites should be made. Review of cultures obtained is also necessary.

When organisms are identified, additional codes should be applied. Consider querying the QHCP if the results of the culture support an organism type but the QHCP's documentation does not list the organism and its connection to the infected site.

Skin ulcers occur for several reasons. For example, disease processes may cause skin ulcers. Common types are cellulitis associated, diabetic, arteriosclerotic, and venous. External factors can also produce ulceration of the skin. Pressure or decubitus ulcers are formed when extreme pressure or an extended period of continuous pressure is placed on the skin and its underlying tissue. These ulcers often occur near bony prominences. Patients with limited mobility are more at risk for development of these types of ulcers.

Patients with sensory impairment to the affected area may not realize that a skin ulcer is occurring due to inability to sense pain properly.

Patients with diabetes are more susceptible to skin ulcers, especially of the feet, but the coder should not assume that all skin ulcers in a diabetic patient are diabetic ulcers. A query should be generated when the cause or type of skin ulcer is not identified.

With pressure or decubitus skin ulcers, the stage or qualifying descriptors must also be noted in the record. Only the pressure or decubitus ulcer requires staging or qualifying descriptors, however; other forms of skin ulcers are not classified by this staging process.

Specific coding guidelines note that once the QHCP has identified the ulcer, type, and location, further staging or qualifying descriptors can be taken from the documentation of health care providers that have been identified by a facility to further provide staging or qualifying descriptors.

Review of coding guidelines and *Coding Clinic* on this subject is vital to the coder when preparing a coding abstract for a chart with decubitus or pressure ulcer documentation. When no documentation of the stage or qualifying descriptors is found within the record, a query should be written to the QHCP. Appendix C will provide the coder with insight on how to generate a query.

When the QHCP does not state the cause or type of ulcer, the coder should be careful not to assume linkage to a stated disease. It is the responsibility of the QHCP to state this cause.

Based on the provided inpatient setting documentation, please assign the following:

- MS-DRG assignment
- ICD-9-CM diagnosis codes (FY2010)
- POA indicators

| MS-DRG Assignment | | | |
|---|---|---|---|

| ICD-9-CM Diagnosis Codes | ICD-9-CM Diagnosis Description | POA | Coding Clinic Reference/Reason |
|---|---|---|---|
| | | | |
| | | | |
| | | | |
| | | | |
| | | | |
| | | | |
| | | | |
| | | | |
| | | | |
| | | | |

| Query for QHCP |
|---|
| |

# ADVANCED HEALTH RECORD

The health records of patients who present to the hospital after suffering a traumatic injury to a limb require a thorough review of not only the site(s) affected but also the patient's overall health condition. When a foreign object traumatically enters a limb, it can introduce organisms to the body that can lead to infections, leave small foreign particles behind after its removal, and cause injury to all body parts it has entered.

The QHCP will assess the patient for signs and symptoms of infection, both localized and systemic. Review of the sepsis sections of appendixes A and B will assist the coder in knowing when to consider an infectious process as systemic.

Even though the puncture site can be small, as in the case of a nail puncture, the coder should review the record for documentation of infection in surrounding tissue as well as in structures beneath the puncture site. Cellulitis, abscesses, and osteomyelitis are common types of infection with this kind of injury.

The skin, subcutaneous tissue, muscle, tendons, blood vessels, nerves, and bone structures are all assessed for potential injury. Review of radiology reports such as x-rays, CAT scans, and MRIs will assist the coder in ensuring that all injuries have been documented by the QHCP.

When the organism has been identified by the QHCP, the coder should apply additional codes for all organisms involved. Remember that the QHCP needs to identify in his or her documentation the organism responsible for the infection. The coder cannot apply codes based on the culture reports' documentation until it has been attested to by the QHCP within his or her documentation. A query should be generated if this documentation is not found. Appendix C will provide the coder with assistance in the querying process.

Treatment of infection will usually involve antibiotics as well as possible incision and drainage and/or debridement. Distinct coding guidelines and rules are pertinent depending on what type of debridement is performed. The QHCP must state that the debridement was excisional before the coder can apply a code for excisional debridement, for example.

An excisional debridement involves the use of a sharp or cutting device that removes more than mere loose fragments of tissue. The removal of tissue should be deep enough so that viable tissue has been reached. This activity should be described within the procedure note. It is important to code to the deepest structure debrided. Coding guidelines and *Coding Clinic* related to these procedures should be reviewed thoroughly.

The patient's overall health condition may greatly affect the healing process. Disease processes may slow the body's ability to heal, as may a patient's substance abuse or state of malnutrition.

Based on the provided inpatient setting documentation, please assign the following:

- MS-DRG assignment
- ICD-9-CM diagnosis and procedure codes (FY2010)
- POA indicators

| MS-DRG Assignment |
|---|
|  |

| ICD-9-CM Diagnosis Codes | ICD-9-CM Diagnosis Description | POA | Coding Clinic Reference/Reason |
|---|---|---|---|
|  |  |  |  |
|  |  |  |  |
|  |  |  |  |
|  |  |  |  |
|  |  |  |  |
|  |  |  |  |
|  |  |  |  |
|  |  |  |  |
|  |  |  |  |
|  |  |  |  |
|  |  |  |  |
|  |  |  |  |
|  |  |  |  |
|  |  |  |  |

| ICD-9-CM Procedure Codes | ICD-9-CM Procedure Description |
|---|---|
| | |
| | |
| | |
| | |
| | |

# Endocrine, Nutritional and Metabolic Diseases and Disorders

# BASIC HEALTH RECORD

Hyponatremia has numerous causes. When a patient presents with this condition, the QHCP will review the patient's current diseases and disorders, the patient's medication regimen, and the recent chain of events to try to determine the cause of this electrolyte imbalance.

Often, this is a process of elimination. It is not uncommon, when reviewing the record, to see a list of possible causes documented at the time of admission. Throughout the hospital course, a battery of tests, treatments, and reviews will be conducted to establish the underlying cause. The final determination of the cause may factor into determining the principal diagnosis. The electrolyte imbalance itself may well become the principal diagnosis, or it may be the underlying disease or condition that is determined to be the principal. Only through diligent review of the QHCP's documentation will the coder be able to make this determination.

Depending on the severity of the hyponatremia, the more common presenting signs include headache, malaise, nausea, altered mental status, decreased reflexes, and possible seizure activity. The coder should, however, be cautious when reviewing charts not to assume that all symptoms are linked to just one diagnosis. Often, a patient's presenting symptoms will all have different underlying causes. Similarly, a symptom may be linked to more than one condition. For example, a patient may present with syncope and subsequently be diagnosed with hypovolemia, electrolyte imbalances, or a subdural hemorrhage, but these conditions are not necessarily the cause of the syncope. Review of the syncope section in appendix A and the CVA sections in appendixes A and B may provide insight into these types of conditions.

Only the QHCP can make the linkage between the symptoms and the cause. When symptoms do not have a stated cause, they should continue to be identified separately through the coding abstract.

Based on the provided inpatient setting documentation, please assign the following:

- MS-DRG assignment
- ICD-9-CM diagnosis and procedure codes (FY2010)
- POA indicators

| MS-DRG Assignment |
|---|
|  |

| ICD-9-CM Diagnosis Codes | ICD-9-CM Diagnosis Description | POA | Coding Clinic Reference/Reason |
|---|---|---|---|
|  |  |  |  |
|  |  |  |  |
|  |  |  |  |
|  |  |  |  |
|  |  |  |  |
|  |  |  |  |
|  |  |  |  |
|  |  |  |  |
|  |  |  |  |
|  |  |  |  |
|  |  |  |  |
|  |  |  |  |
|  |  |  |  |
|  |  |  |  |

| ICD-9-CM Procedure Codes | ICD-9-CM Procedure Description |
|---|---|
|  |  |
|  |  |
|  |  |
|  |  |
|  |  |

## INTERMEDIATE HEALTH RECORD

A patient may present to the hospital setting with DKA without an already-established diagnosis of diabetes. In fact, it is not uncommon for this acute condition to be the first noticeable sign of diabetes. Established diabetic patients can also develop this condition when the disease is not under control.

Several coding guidelines and *Coding Clinic* are pertinent to the subject of diabetes and should be reviewed.

When a patient does not produce his or her own insulin to convert glucose (sugar) into energy, he or she will start to burn stored fat for energy use. By-products of this fat consumption are called ketones. The body will also have increased acid production. The term *ketoacidosis* is derived from these two by-products.

When large amounts of fat are burned, ketones can be found in the urine, and acid levels in the blood will increase. Patients may present with complaints of fatigue, muscle stiffness, fruity mouth odor, excessive thirst, increased urination, nausea, vomiting, and shortness of breath with increased respiratory rate.

Ketones found in the urine, acidosis, and several different types of electrolyte imbalances are common clinical signs of DKA. Blood glucose levels will be extremely elevated. If not detected early, mental status changes will arise, progressing to encephalopathy and coma if DKA is not treated promptly. Organ failures and infarctions may also occur when DKA becomes advanced. Acute renal failure, myocardial infarctions, bowel infarctions, and cerebral edema are examples of more advanced effects of DKA. The renal failure section of appendix A and the CVA and MI sections of appendix B will assist the coder in identifying these advanced conditions.

The coder should review the record closely for all electrolyte imbalances as well as for diagnoses resulting from affected organs. Acuity of these organ dysfunctions, failures, and infarctions should be identified by the QHCP. A query should be considered when the acuity is not identified. Appendix C is a useful tool for query formatting.

Based on the provided inpatient setting documentation, please assign the following:

- MS-DRG assignment
- ICD-9-CM diagnosis codes (FY2010)
- POA indicators

*ICD-9-CM and POA Coding Mentor,* edited by Patricia L. Bower-Jernigan, RHIA.

| MS-DRG Assignment |
|---|
|  |

| ICD-9-CM Diagnosis Codes | ICD-9-CM Diagnosis Description | POA | Coding Clinic Reference/Reason |
|---|---|---|---|
|  |  |  |  |
|  |  |  |  |
|  |  |  |  |
|  |  |  |  |
|  |  |  |  |
|  |  |  |  |
|  |  |  |  |
|  |  |  |  |
|  |  |  |  |
|  |  |  |  |

| Query for QHCP |
|---|
|  |

# ADVANCED HEALTH RECORD

It is essential when coding records with a presenting symptom of chest pain to pay close attention to the QHCP's documentation for a final determination of what caused this symptom. While chest pain is often associated with cardiovascular disease, it can also occur with numerous other conditions or diseases. Usually, the QHCP will order testing to rule out cardiovascular conditions first. If AMI is determined to be the cause of the chest pain, it must be dealt with promptly, as it is a life-threatening condition.

When cardiovascular diagnoses are ruled out, the QHCP will begin assessing for other commonly associated diagnoses. The type of treatment needed to alleviate the chest pain is generally further explored. This is a process of elimination, by way of treatment plans and a variety of tests.

While diabetes is not usually the first diagnosis associated with chest pain, it can have this presenting feature. When diabetes is out of control, the stress on the body can manifest itself in several ways. Reviewing the record thoroughly will help the coder find the determined cause of the chest pain. If the cause is not concisely documented, the coder should generate a query to the QHCP for clarification.

A query appears within this health record. Since the time of its writing, more stringent guidelines have been established for the query process. Appendix C will assist the coder with this process.

Based on the provided inpatient setting documentation, please assign the following:

- MS-DRG assignment
- ICD-9-CM diagnosis and procedure codes (FY2010)
- POA indicators

*ICD-9-CM and POA Coding Mentor*, edited by Patricia L. Bower-Jernigan, RHIA.

| | MS-DRG Assignment | | |
|---|---|---|---|

| ICD-9-CM Diagnosis Codes | ICD-9-CM Diagnosis Description | POA | Coding Clinic Reference/Reason |
|---|---|---|---|
| | | | |
| | | | |
| | | | |
| | | | |
| | | | |
| | | | |
| | | | |
| | | | |
| | | | |
| | | | |
| | | | |
| | | | |
| | | | |
| | | | |
| | | | |

| ICD-9-CM Procedure Codes | ICD-9-CM Procedure Description |
|---|---|
| | |
| | |
| | |
| | |
| | |
| | |
| | |
| | |
| | |
| | |

# Diseases and Disorders
# of the Kidney and Urinary Tract

## BASIC HEALTH RECORD

When patients present with an acute infectious process, review all clinical data, including laboratory results, vital signs, x-rays, scans, and any additional studies, to determine whether any evidence indicates a more specified diagnosis or a systemic illness associated with an infectious process. The section on urinary tract infection in appendix A and the sections on sepsis in appendixes A, B, and C will help guide the coder in determining when it is appropriate to query the QHCP for more specified diagnoses in this scenario.

The category of infectious process known as SIRS generally refers to the body's physiological response to infection, trauma, burns, or other insults such as cancer or pancreatitis. The symptoms can include fever, leukocytosis, tachycardia, and tachypnea.

Sepsis is generally referred to as SIRS due to an infection. When evidence within a record indicates additional or more specified diagnoses, it is appropriate for the coder to query the QHCP. For assistance in the query process, see appendix C.

The coder needs to be diligent in review of the health record, as at times diagnoses will be listed that are not relevant to the current encounter. All documented secondary diagnoses must meet one of the five criteria for reporting additional diagnoses as outlined in the general coding guidelines on reporting additional diagnoses: (1) clinical evaluation, (2) therapeutic treatment, (3) diagnostic procedures, (4) extended length of hospital stay, and (5) increased nursing care and/or monitoring. These criteria should be considered for each secondary diagnosis. If one or more of these criteria are met, then the secondary diagnosis should be coded. However, if none of these five criteria is met, the secondary diagnosis listed should be excluded from the coding

Based on the provided inpatient setting documentation, please assign the following:

- MS-DRG assignment
- ICD-9-CM diagnosis and procedure codes (FY2010)
- POA indicators

| MS-DRG Assignment |
|---|
| |

| ICD-9-CM Diagnosis Codes | ICD-9-CM Diagnosis Description | POA | Coding Clinic Reference/Reason |
|---|---|---|---|
| | | | |
| | | | |
| | | | |
| | | | |
| | | | |
| | | | |
| | | | |
| | | | |
| | | | |
| | | | |

| ICD-9-CM Procedure Codes | ICD-9-CM Procedure Description |
|---|---|
|  |  |
|  |  |
|  |  |
|  |  |
|  |  |

| Query for QHCP |
|---|
|  |

## INTERMEDIATE HEALTH RECORD

When coding, certain signs and symptom codes should not be applied to the abstract if they are considered integral to the disease process, as in the case of hematuria with kidney stones. Because hematuria is integral to the disease process of kidney stones, it would not be coded as an additional secondary diagnosis. In contrast, some secondary diagnoses should be added when they are not routinely associated with the disease. See *Coding Clinic* and coding guidelines for clarification of this type of situation.

Review the record for additional secondary diagnoses, as they can be reflective of the patient's medical condition in its entirety. Sometimes, the MS-DRG, the severity of illness, or the risk of mortality will be affected by secondary diagnoses.

Based on the provided inpatient setting documentation, please assign the following:

- MS-DRG assignment
- ICD-9-CM diagnosis and procedure codes (FY2010)
- POA indicators

*ICD-9-CM and POA Coding Mentor,* edited by Patricia L. Bower-Jernigan, RHIA.

| MS-DRG Assignment |
|---|
| |

| ICD-9-CM Diagnosis Codes | ICD-9-CM Diagnosis Description | POA | Coding Clinic Reference/Reason |
|---|---|---|---|
| | | | |
| | | | |
| | | | |
| | | | |
| | | | |
| | | | |
| | | | |
| | | | |
| | | | |
| | | | |

| ICD-9-CM Procedure Codes | ICD-9-CM Procedure Description |
|---|---|
|  |  |
|  |  |
|  |  |
|  |  |
|  |  |

| Query for QHCP |
|---|
|  |

*ICD-9-CM and POA Coding Mentor,* edited by Patricia L. Bower-Jernigan, RHIA.

# ADVANCED HEALTH RECORD

Frequently, more than one diagnosis is present, evaluated, and treated upon a patient's admission to the hospital. Careful inspection of the entire health record is required to determine which diagnosis should be designated as the principal diagnosis. The coder must refer to coding guidelines when selecting the most appropriate principal diagnosis.

When a source of infection is revealed in the documentation from the QHCP and the patient has clinical indicators suggesting SIRS, it is appropriate for the coder to query the QHCP for clarification. The SIRS condition is the body's physiological response to infection, trauma, burns, or other insults such as cancer or pancreatitis. The clinical indicators can include fever, leukocytosis, tachycardia, and tachypnea. When these indicators are seen, the coder can refer to the sepsis sections of appendixes A and B. The pneumonia sections in appendixes A and B can be used as a resource when a diagnosis of pneumonia is made. They will guide the coder in writing a query when a more specified pneumonia type is suspected or questioned. See appendix C for further guidance in the query process.

Once all data are reviewed and the QHCP has responded to the queries, the coder will be able to make a decision, after careful review, as to which diagnosis should be deemed the principal diagnosis.

Based on the provided inpatient setting documentation, please assign the following:

- MS-DRG assignment
- ICD-9-CM diagnosis and procedure codes (FY2010)
- POA indicators

| MS-DRG Assignment |
|---|
| |

| ICD-9-CM Diagnosis Codes | ICD-9-CM Diagnosis Description | POA | Coding Clinic Reference/Reason |
|---|---|---|---|
| | | | |
| | | | |
| | | | |
| | | | |
| | | | |
| | | | |
| | | | |
| | | | |
| | | | |
| | | | |
| | | | |
| | | | |
| | | | |
| | | | |
| | | | |

(Continued on next page)

| ICD-9-CM Diagnosis Codes | ICD-9-CM Diagnosis Description | POA | Coding Clinic Reference/Reason |
|---|---|---|---|
| | | | |
| | | | |
| | | | |
| | | | |

| ICD-9-CM Procedure Codes | ICD-9-CM Procedure Description |
|---|---|
| | |
| | |
| | |
| | |
| | |

| Query for QHCP |
|---|
| |

| Query for QHCP |
|---|
| |

# Diseases and Disorders
# of the Male Reproductive System

## BASIC HEALTH RECORD

The condition known as BPH is caused by increased cell production that leads to enlargement of the prostate. This enlargement can affect males' ability to eliminate urine. In the diagnosis process, a change in the urine stream flow is noted. The patient's health record may describe his symptoms as a weak urine stream flow, interrupted flow, or an increase in frequency and urgency. Patients may also exhibit urine leakage between voiding.

Although BPH is not a form of cancer, its symptoms can be seen in prostate cancer as well. Patients are prompted to seek medical attention when these symptoms occur.

Coding guidelines and *Coding Clinic* indicate those symptoms of BPH that are included in the codes for BPH and those that should be coded separately. A thorough review of these guidelines and *Coding Clinic* will assist the coder in proper code assignments.

Several treatment options are available for patients with BPH. Transurethral prostatectomy is a very common procedure for correction of this condition. Because the condition involves cell production, patients may experience recurrences of BPH after initial treatment.

Based on the provided inpatient setting documentation, please assign the following:

- MS-DRG assignment
- ICD-9-CM diagnosis and procedure codes (FY2010)
- POA indicators

| MS-DRG Assignment | | | |
|---|---|---|---|
| | | | |

| ICD-9-CM Diagnosis Codes | ICD-9-CM Diagnosis Description | POA | Coding Clinic Reference/Reason |
|---|---|---|---|
| | | | |
| | | | |
| | | | |
| | | | |
| | | | |
| | | | |
| | | | |
| | | | |
| | | | |
| | | | |

| ICD-9-CM Procedure Codes | ICD-9-CM Procedure Description |
|---|---|
| | |
| | |
| | |
| | |
| | |

## INTERMEDIATE HEALTH RECORD

A radical prostatectomy involves the removal of not only the prostate itself but also the supporting glands. It may also involve the removal of the surrounding lymph nodes. It is important for the coder to review coding guidelines and *Coding Clinic* to determine which procedures are coded as included in a radical prostatectomy and which procedures take separate codes.

A radical prostatectomy is usually preformed in the presence of known or suspected prostate cancer. It is imperative that the coder review the pathology report to ensure that the QHCP has documented the results in the progress note or discharge summary. Pathology results can only be coded once the QHCP has attested to them.

Careful review of the preoperative and postoperative conditions will allow the coder to capture the correct secondary diagnoses for the coding abstract. The coder should be mindful of the coding guidelines related to reporting a secondary diagnosis. All documented secondary diagnoses must meet one of the following five criteria as outlined in the general coding guidelines on reporting additional diagnoses: (1) clinical evaluation, (2) therapeutic treatment, (3) diagnostic procedures, (4) extended length of hospital stay, and (5) increased nursing care and/or monitoring. Each criterion should be considered for each secondary diagnosis. If one or more of these criteria are met, then the secondary diagnosis should be coded. However, if none of these five criteria is met, the secondary diagnosis listed should be excluded from the coding.

Based on the provided inpatient setting documentation, please assign the following:

- MS-DRG assignment
- ICD-9-CM diagnosis and procedure codes (FY2010)
- POA indicators

| MS-DRG Assignment | | | |
|---|---|---|---|

| ICD-9-CM Diagnosis Codes | ICD-9-CM Diagnosis Description | POA | Coding Clinic Reference/Reason |
|---|---|---|---|
|  |  |  |  |
|  |  |  |  |
|  |  |  |  |
|  |  |  |  |
|  |  |  |  |
|  |  |  |  |
|  |  |  |  |
|  |  |  |  |
|  |  |  |  |
|  |  |  |  |

| ICD-9-CM Procedure Codes | ICD-9-CM Procedure Description |
|---|---|
|  |  |
|  |  |
|  |  |
|  |  |
|  |  |

## ADVANCED HEALTH RECORD

With advances in medical technology expanding, the treatment options for prostate cancer continue to increase. Robot-assisted procedures are becoming more prevalent in the operating room. Robotic applications perform a less invasive procedure, which can result in a shorter length of stay in the hospital and fewer complications following the procedure.

Despite the improved outcomes related to these advances, careful review of the patient's health record should still be conducted for documentation of comorbidities and complications. With patients who have existing conditions that affect the respiratory system, such as COPD, asthma, and obstructive sleep apnea, the coder should vigilantly examine the documentation for indication of respiratory distress following surgery. Anesthesia's effects on these patient types can lead to postsurgery respiratory compromise.

Based on the provided inpatient setting documentation, please assign the following:

- MS-DRG assignment
- ICD-9-CM diagnosis and procedure codes (FY2010)
- POA indicators

| MS-DRG Assignment |
|---|
| |

| ICD-9-CM Diagnosis Codes | ICD-9-CM Diagnosis Description | POA | Coding Clinic Reference/Reason |
|---|---|---|---|
| | | | |
| | | | |
| | | | |
| | | | |
| | | | |
| | | | |
| | | | |
| | | | |
| | | | |
| | | | |
| | | | |
| | | | |
| | | | |
| | | | |

| ICD-9-CM Procedure Codes | ICD-9-CM Procedure Description |
|---|---|
|  |  |
|  |  |
|  |  |
|  |  |
|  |  |

# CHAPTER 13

# Diseases and Disorders of the Female Reproductive System

## BASIC HEALTH RECORD

When a patient is admitted to the hospital for surgery, it is prudent for the coder to review the complete health record for the most detailed descriptions of the diagnoses and procedure.

In the case of women who are treated surgically for benign tumors of the smooth muscle of the uterus, called leiomyomas, the pathology report may be unavailable to the QHCP at the time of discharge. It is appropriate for the coder to query the provider for the pathology results (primary site and any metastatic sites) to obtain the greatest specificity possible. See appendix C for assistance in the writing of queries.

Careful examination of the record is essential for applying all secondary codes to depict an accurate and thorough representation of the patient and the events of the hospital stay.

When applying codes for obesity, morbid obesity, or underweight, certain V codes reflect the BMI of patients. The V code, along with a diagnosis indicating weight status, should be added to the coding abstract. The diagnosis indicating weight status must be documented by a QHCP, whereas the BMI can be documented and coded from a dietitian's note, as he or she is considered an established QHCP.

Based on the provided inpatient setting documentation, please assign the following:

- MS-DRG assignment
- ICD-9-CM diagnosis and procedure codes (FY2010)
- POA indicators

| MS-DRG Assignment |
| --- |
|  |

| ICD-9-CM Diagnosis Codes | ICD-9-CM Diagnosis Description | POA | Coding Clinic Reference/Reason |
| --- | --- | --- | --- |
|  |  |  |  |
|  |  |  |  |
|  |  |  |  |
|  |  |  |  |
|  |  |  |  |

| ICD-9-CM Procedure Codes | ICD-9-CM Procedure Description |
| --- | --- |
|  |  |
|  |  |
|  |  |
|  |  |
|  |  |

| Query for QHCP |
| --- |
|  |

*ICD-9-CM and POA Coding Mentor,* edited by Patricia L. Bower-Jernigan, RHIA.

# INTERMEDIATE HEALTH RECORD

Each year many women are treated for problems related to uterovaginal prolapse, stress urinary incontinence, and vaginal enteroceles. These patients can experience discomfort, pressure, and embarrassment due to urinary incontinence and thus seek treatment, which can include surgery.

The coder must carefully examine the health record to apply the most specific diagnosis and procedure codes related to the encounter he or she is reviewing. Numerous procedures may be performed for these patients in an effort to achieve the best possible repair and fixation.

Review *Coding Clinic* and coding guidelines to assist in proper code selection for these procedures.

Based on the provided inpatient setting documentation, please assign the following:

- MS-DRG assignment
- ICD-9-CM diagnosis and procedure codes (FY2010)
- POA indicators

## MS-DRG Assignment

| ICD-9-CM Diagnosis Codes | ICD-9-CM Diagnosis Description | POA | Coding Clinic Reference/Reason |
|---|---|---|---|
| | | | |
| | | | |
| | | | |
| | | | |
| | | | |

| ICD-9-CM Procedure Codes | ICD-9-CM Procedure Description |
|---|---|
|  |  |
|  |  |
|  |  |
|  |  |
|  |  |
|  |  |
|  |  |
|  |  |
|  |  |
|  |  |

## ADVANCED HEALTH RECORD

It is essential in achieving accurate code assignment to determine the principal diagnosis after study. If the documentation of the pathology report lacks specificity as to primary or secondary sites of malignancy, it is appropriate for the coder to request clarification from the QHCP.

Specific coding guidelines and *Coding Clinic* address malignancies as well as invasive or metastatic sites. It is prudent for the coder to review all laboratory results and pathology reports for any additional diagnoses or findings that may need clarification from the QHCP.

Ovarian cancer can be fairly asymptomatic until it has spread extensively. The symptoms can include abdominal pain or bloating, early satiety (feeling full after eating a small amount of food), and frequent urination. Because patients do not typically consider these symptoms to be alarming, their disease is often extensive before they seek treatment.

After reading the documentation of the providers, if the coder is unable to gain an understanding of whether a diagnosis is current, resolved, or strictly a history of a disease process, then it is proper to clarify the diagnosis by querying the QHCP. For guidelines on writing a query, see appendix C.

Based on the provided inpatient setting documentation, please assign the following:

- MS-DRG assignment
- ICD-9-CM diagnosis and procedure codes (FY2010)
- POA indicators

*ICD-9-CM and POA Coding Mentor,* edited by Patricia L. Bower-Jernigan, RHIA.
Copyright ©2010 Health Forum, Inc., an American Hospital Association company. All rights reserved.

| MS-DRG Assignment | | | |
| --- | --- | --- | --- |

| ICD-9-CM Diagnosis Codes | ICD-9-CM Diagnosis Description | POA | Coding Clinic Reference/Reason |
| --- | --- | --- | --- |
|  |  |  |  |
|  |  |  |  |
|  |  |  |  |
|  |  |  |  |
|  |  |  |  |
|  |  |  |  |
|  |  |  |  |
|  |  |  |  |
|  |  |  |  |
|  |  |  |  |

| ICD-9-CM Procedure Codes | ICD-9-CM Procedure Description |
|---|---|
|  |  |
|  |  |
|  |  |
|  |  |
|  |  |

| Query for QHCP |
|---|
|  |

| Query for QHCP |
|---|
|  |

*ICD-9-CM and POA Coding Mentor,* edited by Patricia L. Bower-Jernigan, RHIA.

# Pregnancy, Childbirth and the Puerperium

## BASIC HEALTH RECORD

When reviewing records of women who are hospitalized for labor and delivery, it is necessary for the coder to consult the coding guidelines and *Coding Clinic* to gain an understanding of how to select the principal diagnosis for each encounter.

Different guidelines exist for this patient population in regard to code selection and the impact of any diagnosis on the patient and the pregnancy. The coder needs a basic understanding of the normal events that occur during labor and delivery to be able to detect when an abnormal event occurs.

In the event that a birth occurs, the coding abstract of the mother will have a V code assigned to it indicating the outcome of a birth.

When a patient is admitted to the hospital and her baby is in the breech position, it is possible that attempts will be made to rotate the baby's position to allow for a vaginal delivery. When rotation cannot be done, most often the mother will have the baby delivered via Cesarean section to avoid complications affecting the infant.

Based on the provided inpatient setting documentation, please assign the following:

- MS-DRG assignment
- ICD-9-CM diagnosis and procedure codes (FY2010)
- POA indicators

| MS-DRG Assignment |
|---|
|  |

| ICD-9-CM Diagnosis Codes | ICD-9-CM Diagnosis Description | POA | Coding Clinic Reference/Reason |
|---|---|---|---|
|  |  |  |  |
|  |  |  |  |
|  |  |  |  |
|  |  |  |  |
|  |  |  |  |

| ICD-9-CM Procedure Codes | ICD-9-CM Procedure Description |
|---|---|
|  |  |
|  |  |
|  |  |
|  |  |
|  |  |

# INTERMEDIATE HEALTH RECORD

Reviewing *Coding Clinic* and coding guidelines for pregnancy, childbirth, and the puerperium is essential for the coder to gain insight into the proper principal diagnosis selection for each individual case.

In some cases, the complication (if any) of the delivery becomes the principal diagnosis. Furthermore, certain codes are added to the mother's coding abstract that are indicative of the status of the infant.

Pregnant women are tested to determine if they are carriers of group B *streptococcus*. A positive test indicates the woman is a carrier, not the existence of an infection. To prevent complications to the infant in such a case, antibiotics are administered to the mother during labor and delivery. Consult the coding guidelines and *Coding Clinic* to assist coding in this situation.

The coder is responsible for reading the procedure notes and assigning those codes for procedures conducted during the hospital encounter that are required by his or her facility.

Based on the provided inpatient setting documentation, please assign the following:

- MS-DRG assignment
- ICD-9-CM diagnosis and procedure codes (FY2010)
- POA indicators

| MS-DRG Assignment | | | |
| --- | --- | --- | --- |

| ICD-9-CM Diagnosis Codes | ICD-9-CM Diagnosis Description | POA | Coding Clinic Reference/Reason |
| --- | --- | --- | --- |
| | | | |
| | | | |
| | | | |
| | | | |
| | | | |
| | | | |
| | | | |
| | | | |
| | | | |
| | | | |

| ICD-9-CM Procedure Codes | ICD-9-CM Procedure Description |
|---|---|
| | |
| | |
| | |
| | |
| | |

## ADVANCED HEALTH RECORD

Cervical incompetence is a condition in which a woman's cervix begins to thin and dilate before the pregnancy reaches full term. The result can be premature dilation of the cervix and premature birth. Cervical incompetence is different from premature labor in that the cervix dilates as a result of pressure and weight of the uterus and infant rather than from contractions. In some cases, sutures are placed in the cervix to strengthen the muscle; this surgical procedure is referred to as a cerclage. A cerclage is performed by a QHCP and actually narrows the cervical opening, the goal being to prevent the cervix from dilating and thereby preventing premature births.

Any record can contain conflicting information. If this occurs, it is appropriate for the coder to query the attending QHCP as to what diagnosis is most accurate for this patient for the current encounter. See appendix C for guidelines in writing a query.

Be cautious in review of documentation that includes a QHCP's use of "watch for." This phrase is meant to indicate that a diagnosis may occur and that the provider is being mindful to be observant for its occurrence. Review of the laboratory results or the clinical indicators for the diagnosis for which the QHCP is watching will assist the coder in determining if indeed it has occurred. The watch-for diagnosis should not be coded if it has not occurred.

Based on the provided inpatient setting documentation, please assign the following:

- MS-DRG assignment
- ICD-9-CM diagnosis and procedure codes (FY2010)
- POA indicators

*ICD-9-CM and POA Coding Mentor,* edited by Patricia L. Bower-Jernigan, RHIA.

| | MS-DRG Assignment | | |
|---|---|---|---|

| ICD-9-CM Diagnosis Codes | ICD-9-CM Diagnosis Description | POA | Coding Clinic Reference/Reason |
|---|---|---|---|
| | | | |
| | | | |
| | | | |
| | | | |
| | | | |
| | | | |
| | | | |
| | | | |
| | | | |
| | | | |

| ICD-9-CM Procedure Codes | ICD-9-CM Procedure Description |
|---|---|
|  |  |
|  |  |
|  |  |
|  |  |
|  |  |

| Query for QHCP |
|---|
|  |

# CHAPTER 15

# Newborns and Other Neonates with Conditions Originating in the Perinatal Period

# BASIC HEALTH RECORD

Very specific coding guidelines and *Coding Clinic* pertain to newborn records. The coder must review these carefully to produce an accurate coding abstract.

Only the newborn record should be used when applying codes for the newborn. It can be tempting to use documentation from the mother's record; however, strict guidelines are in place that oppose this practice.

The query process should be used if clarifications of any conditions or diagnoses are needed for proper coding to take place. Appendix C aids the coder in formatting a query if needed.

The principal diagnosis for a newborn depends on three factors: (1) whether the newborn was alive at time of birth, (2) whether the pregnancy was single or multiple, and (3) where the newborn was born.

To be coded as a live birth, the newborn must have a heartbeat or have a recorded respiration. An Apgar score of 0 recorded on the health record means that neither was present. Be aware that a respiratory rate may be present in the record when intubation and artificial respirations are given, but this induced respiration does not indicate a live birth when attempts to resuscitate fail.

A V code signifying birth is only assigned once in a newborn's record. If the newborn is transferring from another facility, the reason for transfer will be the principal diagnosis.

Maturity level and weight of the newborn should be captured through code assignment. Secondary diagnoses should be captured as long as they meet coding guidelines specific to the newborn. Refer to the "How to Use This Workbook" section for the five criteria for secondary diagnoses.

Based on the provided inpatient setting documentation, please assign the following:

- MS-DRG assignment
- ICD-9-CM diagnosis and procedure codes (FY2010)
- POA indicators

| MS-DRG Assignment |
|---|
|  |

| ICD-9-CM Diagnosis Codes | ICD-9-CM Diagnosis Description | POA | Coding Clinic Reference/Reason |
|---|---|---|---|
|  |  |  |  |
|  |  |  |  |
|  |  |  |  |
|  |  |  |  |
|  |  |  |  |

| ICD-9-CM Procedure Codes | ICD-9-CM Procedure Description |
|---|---|
|  |  |
|  |  |
|  |  |
|  |  |
|  |  |

## INTERMEDIATE HEALTH RECORD

When reviewing a newborn's record, careful attention should be paid to the newborn's first minutes of life. Lower Apgar scores can often indicate complications that may require further code assignments. The Apgar test measures the newborn's activity level, pulse rate, tone, appearance, and respiration rate. Each factor is given a score of 0 to 2, with 2 meaning normal or average. When a low Apgar score is noted, the coder should review the scoring tool to see which area is rated low. This information may indicate a complication.

The coder should review all documentation to seek additional diagnoses for the occurrence of a low Apgar score or gather pertinent data and treatment information to generate a query for explanation of the low score if the coder feels this is warranted. Appendix C aids in formatting a query.

Documentation of the presence of meconium in the amniotic fluid should be captured in the code assignment. Meconium is found in the intestinal tract of full-term newborns. Before or during the birthing process, meconium may be expelled into the amniotic fluid. The presence of meconium in the amniotic fluid can lead to serious complications. For example, meconium can enter the lungs, causing potential infection and respiratory compromise. Generally, when meconium is discovered, the newborn's airway passage will be assessed and suctioned for removal of the meconium. If the QHCP suspects that the meconium may have entered the lungs, deep suctioning will be performed, often through an endotracheal tube. This procedure should also be captured in the coding abstract.

Based on the provided inpatient setting documentation, please assign the following:

• MS-DRG assignment
• ICD-9-CM diagnosis codes (FY2010)
• POA indicators

| MS-DRG Assignment |
| --- |
|  |

| ICD-9-CM Diagnosis Codes | ICD-9-CM Diagnosis Description | POA | Coding Clinic Reference/Reason |
| --- | --- | --- | --- |
|  |  |  |  |
|  |  |  |  |
|  |  |  |  |
|  |  |  |  |
|  |  |  |  |

## ADVANCED HEALTH RECORD

Prematurity of a newborn, of either a single or multiple birth, can potentially involve complications for the newborn(s). The QHCP should document that the newborn is considered premature before a code for prematurity is applied. Assuming that a newborn is premature or mature by his or her gestational age alone is not acceptable per coding guidelines; only the QHCP can determine whether a newborn is premature.

The QHCP assesses not only the gestational age but also the maturity level of many other body systems before determining if prematurity is a diagnosis for a newborn. If no documentation of prematurity or maturity is present in the health record, the coder should consider querying the QHCP for clarification of this matter. Appendix C regarding queries assists in formatting a query.

Low birth weight and feeding problems may be complications of a premature newborn, especially in multiple births. Attention should be paid to documentation on feeding and recorded weights while the newborn was hospitalized.

Jaundice of the newborn, sometimes referred to as neonatal hyperbilirubinemia, occurs when excessive levels of bilirubin are found in the bloodstream. This condition can manifest itself by the appearance of a yellowish color of the skin and eyes. Treatment of newborn jaundice generally includes frequent feeding, to assist in flushing out the excess amounts of bilirubin; phototherapy; and sometimes administration of immunoglobin. Special codes pertaining to the newborn will need to be applied when jaundice is documented.

Based on the provided inpatient setting documentation, please assign the following:

- MS-DRG assignment
- ICD-9-CM diagnosis codes (FY2010)
- POA indicators

| MS-DRG Assignment |
| --- |
|  |

| ICD-9-CM Diagnosis Codes | ICD-9-CM Diagnosis Description | POA | Coding Clinic Reference/Reason |
| --- | --- | --- | --- |
|  |  |  |  |
|  |  |  |  |
|  |  |  |  |
|  |  |  |  |
|  |  |  |  |

# Diseases and Disorders of the Blood and Blood-Forming Organs and Immunological Disorders

# BASIC HEALTH RECORD

Chemotherapy is a common treatment for many forms of cancer. The chemotherapy attempts to destroy cancer cells or slow down the rate of their growth.

Generally, cancer cells are more susceptible to the effects of chemotherapy than are the body's normal cells; however, the body's normal cells also can be affected. Chemotherapy's effect on the normal cells can produce side effects for the patient.

Blood cells can also be affected by chemotherapy. Red blood cells, white blood cells, and platelets are the three main components of blood. The RBCs help carry oxygen to the body. Additional components of RBC are Hgb and Hct. When the levels of these components are low, the patient is noted to have anemia.

The WBCs help the body fight off infections. When the WBC level is low, the patient is noted to have neutropenia. When the patient exhibits fevers with a low WBC, he or she is noted to have neutropenic fever. The presence of the fever indicates a possible infection.

Platelets help the body with clotting of the blood. When the platelet level is low, the patient is noted to have thrombocytopenia.

Patients are commonly hospitalized for any of these conditions. When all three of the patient's blood components are affected, the patient is determined to have pancytopenia. It is the responsibility of the QHCP to identify these conditions by their proper terminology. The coder cannot take it upon himself or herself to diagnose a patient with any of these conditions by reviewing the laboratory results. If further clarification is needed, the coder should format a query to the QHCP. Appendix C should be reviewed for the query process.

Patients may receive transfusions and extra monitoring to watch for complications of decreased levels of the blood components. Patients with these complications may be placed in isolation or on specified precautions to keep them from being exposed to further complications.

Coding guidelines and *Coding Clinic* should be reviewed when coding records noting side effects from chemotherapy. These references will also assist the coder with sequencing of the principal diagnosis.

It is important to understand the relevance of coding secondary diagnoses. Secondary diagnoses affect the hospital stay because of the monitoring, testing, treatment, and amount of extra time spent attending to conditions. It is thus essential to have these diagnoses specified to their greatest degree.

There are several different types and causes of diabetes. Attention should be paid when coding the condition of diabetes to ensure that the correct type or cause is captured through the code assignment. When the QHCP's documentation is contradictory for identifying the type or cause, a query may be necessary.

Based on the provided inpatient setting documentation, please assign the following:

- MS-DRG assignment
- ICD-9-CM diagnosis codes (FY2010)
- POA indicators

| MS-DRG Assignment | | | |
| --- | --- | --- | --- |

| ICD-9-CM Diagnosis Codes | ICD-9-CM Diagnosis Description | POA | Coding Clinic Reference/Reason |
| --- | --- | --- | --- |
| | | | |
| | | | |
| | | | |
| | | | |
| | | | |
| | | | |
| | | | |
| | | | |
| | | | |
| | | | |
| | | | |
| | | | |
| | | | |

**Query for QHCP**

**Query for QHCP**

## INTERMEDIATE HEALTH RECORD

Non-Hodgkin's lymphoma is a form of cancer that affects the lymphatic system. Treatment can involve chemotherapy, immunotherapy, radioimmunotherapy, or possible stem cell or bone marrow transplantation. Patients with this form of cancer are monitored closely in both the inpatient and outpatient settings for developing complications.

When a patient with non-Hodgkin's lymphoma develops fever; decreased levels of blood components such as WBC, RBC, or platelets; or other associated symptoms, admission to the hospital setting may occur for further workup and treatment. These patients have a lowered defense against infections, which can develop quickly if not monitored closely.

It is essential for the coder to review the record for treatment focused around these presenting symptoms. Patients with both a fever and a low WBC are noted as having neutropenic fever. If the underlying cause of the neutropenic fever is identified, the coder should assign a code associated with the cause.

Unless the cancer is being treated or tested directly, the complication is usually the cause of the admission and thus should be considered for the principal diagnosis.

Review of the coding guidelines and *Coding Clinic* will assist with this assignment.

Based on the provided inpatient setting documentation, please assign the following:

- MS-DRG assignment
- ICD-9-CM diagnosis and procedure codes (FY2010)
- POA indicators

| MS-DRG Assignment |
|---|
|  |

| ICD-9-CM Diagnosis Codes | ICD-9-CM Diagnosis Description | POA | Coding Clinic Reference/Reason |
|---|---|---|---|
|  |  |  |  |
|  |  |  |  |
|  |  |  |  |
|  |  |  |  |
|  |  |  |  |
|  |  |  |  |
|  |  |  |  |
|  |  |  |  |
|  |  |  |  |
|  |  |  |  |

| ICD-9-CM Procedure Codes | ICD-9-CM Procedure Description |
|---|---|
| | |
| | |
| | |
| | |
| | |

## ADVANCED HEALTH RECORD

Normal RBCs have a disc shape, allowing them to slip easily through the small vessels to deliver oxygen to the body. When a patient has a condition known as sickle-cell disease, the RBCs are misshapen, appearing in a crescent moon shape. This abnormal shape can limit the RBCs' ability to pass easily through the small vessels. They can become clogged within the vessels, causing disruption to the organs. When they inhibit the blood flow to the bone marrow, they can hinder RBC production.

These misshapen RBCs also have a shortened life expectancy. The disruption in blood production coupled with a shortened life expectancy of the RBCs can cause anemia to the patient, who may require transfusions frequently as a result. When patients require frequent or repeated transfusions, iron can build up in the body, causing iron overload.

Patients with sickle-cell disease can experience periods of crisis, which may require hospitalization. These episodes of crisis can be severely painful to the patient. The disease affects several body systems and can lead to lung, bone, kidney, heart, eye, and nervous system disorders or failures.

If the type of disorder is not identified to the extent that the coder feels is needed to assign a specific code, it is important for the coder to query the QHCP for the specificity needed for proper code assignment. Appendix C should be reviewed for help with the querying process.

While coding secondary diagnoses, remember to review appendix B regarding congestive heart failure, which will help identify the different causes of heart failure.

Based on the provided inpatient setting documentation, please assign the following:

- MS-DRG assignment
- ICD-9-CM diagnosis and procedure codes (FY2010)
- POA indicators

| MS-DRG Assignment |
| --- |
|  |

| ICD-9-CM Diagnosis Codes | ICD-9-CM Diagnosis Description | POA | Coding Clinic Reference/Reason |
| --- | --- | --- | --- |
|  |  |  |  |
|  |  |  |  |
|  |  |  |  |
|  |  |  |  |
|  |  |  |  |
|  |  |  |  |
|  |  |  |  |
|  |  |  |  |
|  |  |  |  |
|  |  |  |  |
|  |  |  |  |
|  |  |  |  |
|  |  |  |  |
|  |  |  |  |

| ICD-9-CM Procedure Codes | ICD-9-CM Procedure Description |
|---|---|
|  |  |
|  |  |
|  |  |
|  |  |
|  |  |

| Query for QHCP |
|---|
|  |

| Query for QHCP |
|---|
|  |

# Myeloproliferative Diseases and Disorders and Poorly Differentiated Neoplasms

## BASIC HEALTH RECORD

In the event that a patient is admitted to the hospital strictly for the purpose of receiving chemotherapy, it is appropriate to use a V code as the principal diagnosis. The QHCP should identify within the documentation that the patient is being admitted for this purpose. The malignancy itself will become a secondary diagnosis in cases such as these.

When patients have brain tumors, some secondary diagnoses can be associated with the principal diagnosis. For example, patients often have neurological deficits that may or may not resolve, such as aphasia, weakness, or paralysis. They may also experience seizures, cerebral edema, and visual disturbances.

All documented secondary diagnoses need to meet one of the five criteria for reporting additional diagnoses as outlined in the general coding guidelines on reporting additional diagnoses: (1) clinical evaluation, (2) therapeutic treatment, (3) diagnostic procedures, (4) extended length of hospital stay, and (5) increased nursing care and/or monitoring. Each of these criteria should be considered for each secondary diagnosis. If one or more of these criteria are met, then the secondary diagnosis should be coded. However, if none of these five criteria is met, the secondary diagnosis listed in the patient's health record should be excluded from the coding abstract.

The infusion of chemotherapy is considered a procedure, as is the insertion of an intra-arterial catheterization performed in interventional radiology.

Based on the provided inpatient setting documentation, please assign the following:

* MS-DRG assignment
* ICD-9-CM diagnosis and procedure codes (FY2010)
* POA indicators

| MS-DRG Assignment |
| --- |
|  |

| ICD-9-CM Diagnosis Codes | ICD-9-CM Diagnosis Description | POA | Coding Clinic Reference/Reason |
| --- | --- | --- | --- |
|  |  |  |  |
|  |  |  |  |
|  |  |  |  |
|  |  |  |  |
|  |  |  |  |

| ICD-9-CM Procedure Codes | ICD-9-CM Procedure Description |
| --- | --- |
|  |  |
|  |  |
|  |  |
|  |  |
|  |  |

## INTERMEDIATE HEALTH RECORD

Multiple myeloma is cancer of the plasma cells. Plasma cells are part of the white blood cells. Overproduction of these cells can cause damage to the bones, which causes pain.

This disease is often initially characterized by pain in the bones, excessive fatigue, excessive thirst, and nausea. The patient undergoes several tests to identify the disease as well as to determine how far it has advanced. Once diagnosed, the patient may be treated with chemotherapy, high-dose steroids, stem cell transplantation, and possibly radiation therapy.

Patients with MM are at increased risk of developing infections, anemia, and kidney failure. Specific coding guidelines and *Coding Clinic* have been established for principal diagnosis selection in cases of neoplasms and subsequent complications.

Pancytopenia is a condition in which a combined deficiency of white blood cells, red blood cells, and platelets exists. Specified causes of this condition may require clarification from the QHCP. See appendix C for assistance in formatting a query.

Based on the provided inpatient setting documentation, please assign the following:

- MS-DRG assignment
- ICD-9-CM diagnosis and procedure codes (FY2010)
- POA indicators

| MS-DRG Assignment |
| --- |
|  |

| ICD-9-CM Diagnosis Codes | ICD-9-CM Diagnosis Description | POA | Coding Clinic Reference/Reason |
| --- | --- | --- | --- |
|  |  |  |  |
|  |  |  |  |
|  |  |  |  |
|  |  |  |  |
|  |  |  |  |
|  |  |  |  |
|  |  |  |  |
|  |  |  |  |
|  |  |  |  |
|  |  |  |  |

*ICD-9-CM and POA Coding Mentor,* edited by Patricia L. Bower-Jernigan, RHIA.
Copyright ©2010 Health Forum, Inc., an American Hospital Association company. All rights reserved.

| ICD-9-CM Procedure Codes | ICD-9-CM Procedure Description |
|---|---|
|  |  |
|  |  |
|  |  |
|  |  |
|  |  |

| Query for QHCP |
|---|
|  |

*ICD-9-CM and POA Coding Mentor,* edited by Patricia L. Bower-Jernigan, RHIA.

# ADVANCED HEALTH RECORD

Lymphoma is a cancer that involves the lymph nodes, which are part of the immune system. Presenting symptoms can include painless lumps in the groin, armpits, or neck; fever; night sweats; and fatigue. Symptoms at times are sudden in onset, and the patient can experience somewhat atypical symptoms depending on the location of the lymphoma.

When assigning codes for lymphoma, it is necessary to determine, through the QHCP's documentation, the sites involved. If the documentation within the health record is inadequate, it would be appropriate to query the QHCP. For guidelines in writing a query, see appendix C.

As with any surgical procedure, it is necessary to review the entire operative note for determining the proper procedure codes. Patients who undergo spinal surgeries or have spinal tumors can experience dural tears. If a question arises as to whether a dural tear was a complication of the surgical procedure or a spontaneous occurrence resulting from a tumor, a query should be addressed to the QHCP.

Based on the provided inpatient setting documentation, please assign the following:

- MS-DRG assignment
- ICD-9-CM diagnosis and procedure codes (FY2010)
- POA indicators

| MS-DRG Assignment |
|---|
|  |

| ICD-9-CM Diagnosis Codes | ICD-9-CM Diagnosis Description | POA | Coding Clinic Reference/Reason |
|---|---|---|---|
|  |  |  |  |
|  |  |  |  |
|  |  |  |  |
|  |  |  |  |
|  |  |  |  |
|  |  |  |  |
|  |  |  |  |
|  |  |  |  |
|  |  |  |  |
|  |  |  |  |

| ICD-9-CM Procedure Codes | ICD-9-CM Procedure Description |
|---|---|
|  |  |
|  |  |
|  |  |
|  |  |
|  |  |

| Query for QHCP |
|---|
|  |

| Query for QHCP |
|---|
|  |

*ICD-9-CM and POA Coding Mentor,* edited by Patricia L. Bower-Jernigan, RHIA.

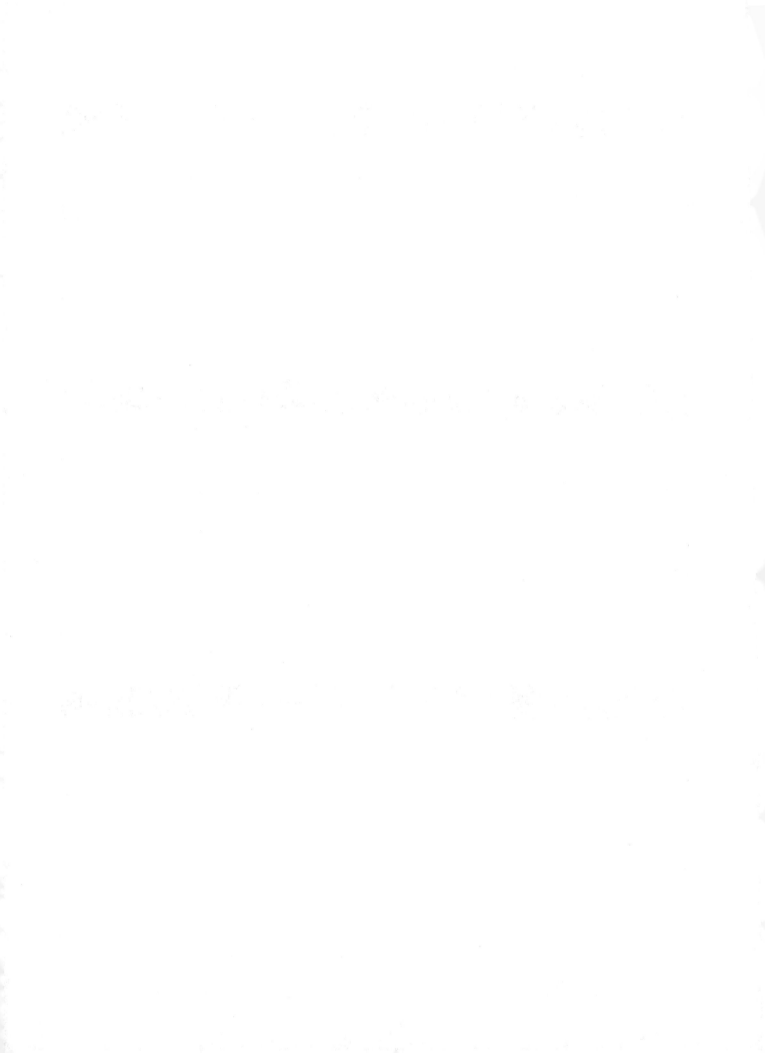

# CHAPTER 18

# Infectious and Parasitic Diseases

# BASIC HEALTH RECORD

Upon admission to the hospital, a patient's health record may show only a list of symptoms as cause for admission. Through a battery of tests, the QHCP will try to identify the cause of the presenting symptoms. A symptom should be replaced by an established or a possible diagnosis once the cause of the symptom has been determined.

Occasions will arise when a possible or an established cause for the symptoms cannot be determined. In this situation, the coder may choose one of the presenting symptoms, and that symptom will be listed as principal diagnosis. All of the other symptoms should be listed as secondary diagnoses.

Based on the provided inpatient setting documentation, please assign the following:

- MS-DRG assignment
- ICD-9-CM diagnosis and procedure codes (FY2010)
- POA indicators

| MS-DRG Assignment |
|---|
|  |

| ICD-9-CM Diagnosis Codes | ICD-9-CM Diagnosis Description | POA | Coding Clinic Reference/Reason |
|---|---|---|---|
|  |  |  |  |
|  |  |  |  |
|  |  |  |  |
|  |  |  |  |
|  |  |  |  |
|  |  |  |  |
|  |  |  |  |
|  |  |  |  |
|  |  |  |  |
|  |  |  |  |

| ICD-9-CM Procedure Codes | ICD-9-CM Procedure Description |
|---|---|
|  |  |
|  |  |
|  |  |
|  |  |
|  |  |

## INTERMEDIATE HEALTH RECORD

Postoperative infections may develop following surgery. When the patient is readmitted to a hospital because of this complication, the coder may need to apply more than one code to describe the condition. The fact that it is a postoperative infection and the infection itself will both need to be captured in the coding.

As specificity is very important in coding, the coder should review the record for the specific organisms causing the infection. If the QHCP has not documented these organisms within the patient documentation but an abnormal culture result is found in the patient's health record, the coder should generate a query for clarification of what organism(s) is presenting with infection and being treated. Appendix C will assist the coder with how to format a query.

A common postoperative infection that occurs following abdominal surgery is an abscess of the abdominal cavity. Patients may exhibit pain at the site, drainage from the incision, and fever. Tests such as CAT scans or MRIs will help identify the presence and the location of the abscess. The QHCP may insert a percutaneous drainage device into the abdominal cavity to allow the abscess to drain. The coder should make sure to capture this intervention through assignment of a procedure code.

Antibiotic treatment most likely will also be ordered. The coder should keep in mind that, when reviewing a health record dealing with any infection, care should be taken to fully evaluate the record for the four elements of SIRS. If the patient exhibits two or more elements in the presence of a known or suspected infection, the coder should determine if a query asking for SIRS and/or sepsis is needed. Review of the sections of appendixes A and B covering sepsis will assist the coder with this determination.

Based on the provided inpatient setting documentation, please assign the following:

- MS-DRG assignment
- ICD-9-CM diagnosis and procedure codes (FY2010)
- POA indicators

*ICD-9-CM and POA Coding Mentor,* edited by Patricia L. Bower-Jernigan, RHIA.

| | MS-DRG Assignment | | |
|---|---|---|---|
| | | | |

| ICD-9-CM Diagnosis Codes | ICD-9-CM Diagnosis Description | POA | Coding Clinic Reference/Reason |
|---|---|---|---|
| | | | |
| | | | |
| | | | |
| | | | |
| | | | |
| | | | |
| | | | |
| | | | |
| | | | |
| | | | |

| ICD-9-CM Procedure Codes | ICD-9-CM Procedure Description |
|---|---|
| | |
| | |
| | |
| | |
| | |

# ADVANCED HEALTH RECORD

When a patient develops a localized infection, the autoimmune system of the body attempts to fight off the infection at the localized area. When an infection is more serious or resistant than the autoimmune system can handle, the body systemically responds to the infection. As a result, SIRS will develop, wherein a patient will exhibit an increase or a decrease in body temperature, an increase in heart rate, an increase in respiratory rate, and an elevation or a decrease in the WBC. When a patient has a known or suspected source of an infection in conjunction with SIRS, sepsis has developed.

Once this systemic process has started, the process can be overwhelming to the body. The body will make every attempt to protect itself and save its vital organs by shutting down body functions. This process is known as organ dysfunction and can be exhibited by acute respiratory failure, myopathy, DIC, encephalopathy, hepatic or liver failure, acute renal failure, and septic shock. The patient would now be considered to have severe sepsis.

Several coding guidelines and *Coding Clinic* pertain to sepsis, severe sepsis, and septic shock. The coder must keep in mind that the QHCP needs to make the linkage between the sepsis and the organ dysfunction before the additional severe sepsis code can be applied. When this diagnosis is unclear, the coder should consider writing a query to the QHCP.

Many QHCPs use terms such as *bacteremia* or *urosepsis* interchangeably with the term *sepsis*. These terms, however, are not equivalent. It is up to the coder to determine if a query for clarification is required to know which diagnosis should be coded.

A systemic illness needs to be sequenced before a localized infection. If the QHCP is documenting bacteremia instead of sepsis or septicemia, the localized infection has to be sequenced first because bacteremia is a symptom code. It is also imperative that the coder identify whether the organism responsible for the localized infection is also responsible for the sepsis.

The sections on sepsis in appendixes A and B further define and provide guidance to understanding the diagnosis of sepsis. The pneumonia sections in appendixes A and B provide clarification on pneumonia types and their associated diagnoses. For further guidance on renal failure, reviewing appendix A may be warranted. Appendix C is a useful tool for assistance with query formatting.

Based on the provided inpatient setting documentation, please assign the following:

- MS-DRG assignment
- ICD-9-CM diagnosis and procedure codes (FY2010)
- POA indicators

| MS-DRG Assignment |
|---|
|  |

| ICD-9-CM Diagnosis Codes | ICD-9-CM Diagnosis Description | POA | Coding Clinic Reference/Reason |
|---|---|---|---|
|  |  |  |  |
|  |  |  |  |
|  |  |  |  |
|  |  |  |  |
|  |  |  |  |
|  |  |  |  |
|  |  |  |  |
|  |  |  |  |
|  |  |  |  |
|  |  |  |  |
|  |  |  |  |
|  |  |  |  |
|  |  |  |  |
|  |  |  |  |

| ICD-9-CM Procedure Codes | ICD-9-CM Procedure Description |
|---|---|
|  |  |
|  |  |
|  |  |
|  |  |
|  |  |

| Query for QHCP |
|---|
|  |

# CHAPTER 19

# Mental Diseases and Disorders

## BASIC HEALTH RECORD

Dysthymic disorder is characterized by chronic depression. This disorder can be seen in children as well as in adults. At times, suicidal ideation will be associated with this disorder. When the patient's health record documents suicidal ideation, it should be added as a V code.

Dysthymic disorder can affect many areas of a person's life, including sleep; appetite; and levels of concentration, self-esteem, and motivation. Treatment can consist of therapy, either individual or group, and antidepressant medications. When diagnoses are listed within the health record that are described as insignificant and required no evaluation, monitoring, or treatment, a code should not be assigned for them on the abstract.

Based on the provided inpatient setting documentation, please assign the following:

- MS-DRG assignment
- ICD-9-CM diagnosis codes (FY2010)
- POA indicators

| | MS-DRG Assignment |
|---|---|
| | |

| ICD-9-CM Diagnosis Codes | ICD-9-CM Diagnosis Description | POA | Coding Clinic Reference/Reason |
|---|---|---|---|
| | | | |
| | | | |
| | | | |
| | | | |
| | | | |

# INTERMEDIATE HEALTH RECORD

The diagnosis of adjustment disorder can have varying features and, depending on the patient, may include more than one component. The QHCP diagnoses the patient mainly by interviewing him or her regarding the events surrounding the current admission and the recent history of stresses the patient has experienced. The goal of treatment is directed at easing the patient's symptoms. Often, individual or group therapy is incorporated into treatment, as are antidepressant or anti-anxiety medications to alleviate the anxiety or depression components that the patient is experiencing.

When diagnoses have occurred prior to the hospitalization that are still under current treatment, evaluation, or monitoring, it is appropriate to assign a corresponding code to capture the diagnosis on the coding abstract.

Based on the provided inpatient setting documentation, please assign the following:

- MS-DRG assignment
- ICD-9-CM diagnosis codes (FY2010)
- POA indicators

| | MS-DRG Assignment | | |
|---|---|---|---|
| | | | |

| ICD-9-CM Diagnosis Codes | ICD-9-CM Diagnosis Description | POA | Coding Clinic Reference/Reason |
|---|---|---|---|
| | | | |
| | | | |
| | | | |
| | | | |
| | | | |
| | | | |
| | | | |
| | | | |
| | | | |
| | | | |
| | | | |
| | | | |
| | | | |
| | | | |

## ADVANCED HEALTH RECORD

Careful review of the entire health record is required when determining the principal diagnosis in the MDC of mental diseases and disorders, as the individual may have several components to his or her diagnosis.

Patients with severe depression or mania and some with schizophrenia are treated with ECT. The procedure involves sedation followed by the passage of electrical current into the brain, evoking a seizure. This procedure affects the brain chemistry and at times provides a quicker form of relief than does medication. Patients undergoing ECT typically require a series of treatment sessions for optimal results.

Based on the provided inpatient setting documentation, please assign the following:

- MS-DRG assignment
- ICD-9-CM diagnosis and procedure codes (FY2010)
- POA indicators

Mental Diseases and Disorders

187

| MS-DRG Assignment | | | |
|---|---|---|---|
|  | | | |

| ICD-9-CM Diagnosis Codes | ICD-9-CM Diagnosis Description | POA | Coding Clinic Reference/Reason |
|---|---|---|---|
|  |  |  |  |
|  |  |  |  |
|  |  |  |  |
|  |  |  |  |
|  |  |  |  |
|  |  |  |  |
|  |  |  |  |
|  |  |  |  |
|  |  |  |  |
|  |  |  |  |
|  |  |  |  |
|  |  |  |  |
|  |  |  |  |
|  |  |  |  |

*ICD-9-CM and POA Coding Mentor,* edited by Patricia L. Bower-Jernigan, RHIA.
Copyright ©2010 Health Forum, Inc., an American Hospital Association company. All rights reserved.

| ICD-9-CM Procedure Codes | ICD-9-CM Procedure Description |
|---|---|
|  |  |
|  |  |
|  |  |
|  |  |
|  |  |

# Alcohol/Drug Use and Alcohol/Drug-Induced Organic Mental Disorders

# BASIC HEALTH RECORD

Alcohol abuse continues to be an ongoing problem in today's society. It can be devastating to the person abusing, his or her family and friends, and society as a whole.

When abuse or excessive alcohol intake is stopped abruptly, alcohol withdrawal can result. Alcohol withdrawal can start within hours of ceasing the alcohol intake or present as late as one to two weeks after cessation. Depending on the severity of the withdrawal, a patient may have behavior or mood changes including depression, excitability, irritability, anxiety, or nervousness. He or she may physically appear jittery or shaky, fatigued, or pale; have clammy skin; or have dilated pupils or abnormal eye movement. Someone experiencing alcohol withdrawal may experience headaches, sweating, a loss of appetite, nausea, and vomiting. His or her sleep may be affected by insomnia or bad dreams, and he or she may lose the ability to react to situations as promptly as is normal for the person.

If withdrawal is allowed to become advanced, the person may develop DTs. A patient with DTs will have confusion and experience visual hallucinations. Convulsions and blackout periods may also occur.

A patient in alcohol withdrawal should be observed closely. Often, such observation will be done in a hospital setting. Close evaluation of the patient's electrolytes and other body systems will be conducted, as will treatment of the exhibited symptoms.

Avoidance of further alcohol intake is the long-term treatment goal. When reviewing a record for alcohol withdrawal, the coder should use the coding guidelines and *Coding Clinic* to help with code assignments and sequencing. It is important to capture in the coding abstract the treatment provided for the patient during the hospital setting. Identify whether both detoxification and rehabilitation have been provided for the patient.

While discharge disposition is a vital element for any coding abstract, the diagnoses pertaining to drug and alcohol abuse will be especially affected by the discharge disposition.

Based on the provided inpatient setting documentation, please assign the following:

- MS-DRG assignment
- ICD-9-CM diagnosis and procedure codes (FY2010)
- POA indicators

| MS-DRG Assignment |
| --- |
|  |

| ICD-9-CM Diagnosis Codes | ICD-9-CM Diagnosis Description | POA | Coding Clinic Reference/Reason |
| --- | --- | --- | --- |
|  |  |  |  |
|  |  |  |  |
|  |  |  |  |
|  |  |  |  |
|  |  |  |  |
|  |  |  |  |
|  |  |  |  |
|  |  |  |  |
|  |  |  |  |
|  |  |  |  |

| ICD-9-CM Procedure Codes | ICD-9-CM Procedure Description |
| --- | --- |
|  |  |
|  |  |
|  |  |
|  |  |
|  |  |

# INTERMEDIATE HEALTH RECORD

Electrolyte imbalances can often accompany alcohol abuse and withdrawal. Alcohol affects the liver and pancreas, which both are vital in the balance of electrolytes in the body.

Absorption and elimination can be affected. Patients tend to lose their appetite during withdrawal and often are noted to be dehydrated.

If electrolyte imbalances are not corrected, they can cause serious complications. For example, hypokalemia can cause arrhythmias of the heart. If hypokalemia is not treated, these arrhythmias can become life threatening.

Another complication, hyponatremia, can cause mental status changes and convulsions. A careful review of the record for these types of conditions should be conducted to ensure an accurate coding abstract is prepared.

Patients who enter the hospital for alcohol withdrawal usually will undergo detoxification as an intervention. This process includes management of the withdrawal symptoms the patient exhibits. In addition to being evaluated and monitored for arising conditions, the patient will receive medicine and nutritional administration. The coder should assign a detoxification code for this intervention.

The patient may also be placed in a rehabilitation program—a structured program that can help the patient abstain from alcohol while providing alternative lifestyle choices. If the rehabilitation program has started during the hospitalization encounter, it is appropriate for the coder to apply a procedure code for this intervention, even if a patient does not stay in the hospital setting for the full program.

When both detoxification and rehabilitation occur, a combination code can be used to capture both of these interventions.

Based on the provided inpatient setting documentation, please assign the following:

- MS-DRG assignment
- ICD-9-CM diagnosis and procedure codes (FY2010)
- POA indicators

| MS-DRG Assignment |
|---|
|  |

| ICD-9-CM Diagnosis Codes | ICD-9-CM Diagnosis Description | POA | Coding Clinic Reference/Reason |
|---|---|---|---|
|  |  |  |  |
|  |  |  |  |
|  |  |  |  |
|  |  |  |  |
|  |  |  |  |
|  |  |  |  |
|  |  |  |  |
|  |  |  |  |
|  |  |  |  |
|  |  |  |  |

| ICD-9-CM Procedure Codes | ICD-9-CM Procedure Description |
|---|---|
|  |  |
|  |  |
|  |  |
|  |  |
|  |  |

## ADVANCED HEALTH RECORD

Complications from alcoholism can be vast. Two frequently seen complications in the hospital setting are pancreatitis and alcoholic hepatitis.

Acute pancreatitis is an inflammation of the pancreas. A patient's serum, urine amylase, and lipase levels will be elevated. The most noted symptom of pancreatitis is the acute pain patients experience; nausea and vomiting are also common. Most patients require pain management through the acute phase as well as bowel rest with administration of intravenous fluids.

Patients with acute alcohol hepatitis will show an elevation in their liver function tests. Symptoms may be absent or subdued, although patients may exhibit a decrease in appetite, nausea, vomiting, fever, jaundice, and even ascites, depending on the severity of the condition. Unless this condition is severe, cessation from alcohol and nutritional support and close monitoring may be all that are needed for treatment.

All secondary diagnoses demonstrated in the alcohol abuse and withdrawal patient need to be evaluated by the coder to determine if they should be added to the coding abstract. Refer to the "How to Use This Workbook" section for the five criteria for secondary diagnoses.

Based on the provided inpatient setting documentation, please assign the following:

- MS-DRG assignment
- ICD-9-CM diagnosis and procedure codes (FY2010)
- POA indicators

| MS-DRG Assignment |
| --- |
| |

| ICD-9-CM Diagnosis Codes | ICD-9-CM Diagnosis Description | POA | Coding Clinic Reference/Reason |
| --- | --- | --- | --- |
| | | | |
| | | | |
| | | | |
| | | | |
| | | | |
| | | | |
| | | | |
| | | | |
| | | | |
| | | | |
| | | | |
| | | | |
| | | | |

| ICD-9-CM Procedure Codes | ICD-9-CM Procedure Description |
|---|---|
|  |  |
|  |  |
|  |  |
|  |  |
|  |  |

# Injury, Poisoning and Toxic Effects of Drugs

# BASIC HEALTH RECORD

Situations arise postoperatively that are considered complications. Patients may be readmitted to the hospital for evaluation, monitoring, and treatment of these conditions.

More than one complication may occur as a result of a surgical procedure. The coder is required to perform a careful review of the documentation of each complication to be able to designate which diagnosis to sequence as the principal diagnosis.

Wound dehiscence, for example, is a condition in which the suture line of an incision opens. This condition can be the result of poor wound healing, which may be attributed to obesity, infection, or too much strain or movement of the suture line. Another example is wound seroma, a condition that can be described as an accumulation of serous fluid within an operative site. Both of these conditions typically require treatment to prevent further problems.

As mentioned, obesity can affect wound healing. The diagnosis of obesity is required to be documented by a QHCP; however, the patient's BMI can be captured from a dietitian's note, as a dietitian is considered a QHCP and thus a source on which to base coding.

When obesity is documented in the health record, the related diagnosis code, and the V code for BMI, should be added for completeness and accuracy.

When a patient is a carrier of MRSA, another potential postoperative complication, a V code should be applied to the coding abstract to indicate this status.

Based on the provided inpatient setting documentation, please assign the following:

- MS-DRG assignment
- ICD-9-CM diagnosis and procedure codes (FY2010)
- POA indicators

| MS-DRG Assignment |
| --- |
| |

| ICD-9-CM Diagnosis Codes | ICD-9-CM Diagnosis Description | POA | Coding Clinic Reference/Reason |
| --- | --- | --- | --- |
| | | | |
| | | | |
| | | | |
| | | | |
| | | | |
| | | | |
| | | | |
| | | | |
| | | | |
| | | | |

| ICD-9-CM Procedure Codes | ICD-9-CM Procedure Description |
| --- | --- |
| | |
| | |
| | |
| | |
| | |

# INTERMEDIATE HEALTH RECORD

When a patient is admitted with gastrointestinal bleeding, the QHCP must determine the source of the bleeding. Documentation in the health record that the bleeding is from a previous surgical site will require assignment of a complication code. If documentation indicates that the bleeding could have been caused by medicinal agents used in therapeutic use, an E code should be applied as well.

The coder should review the patient's laboratory results to determine if any abnormalities were found. If so, and if the coder suspects additional diagnoses apply to the patient, it would be appropriate to query the QHCP using the format established in appendix C.

For patients who have a history of a malignancy or malignancies, it is proper to apply V codes for each site that is documented in the record.

Based on the provided inpatient setting documentation, please assign the following:

*   MS-DRG assignment
*   ICD-9-CM diagnosis codes (FY2010)
*   POA indicators

| MS-DRG Assignment |
| --- |
| |

| ICD-9-CM Diagnosis Codes | ICD-9-CM Diagnosis Description | POA | Coding Clinic Reference/Reason |
| --- | --- | --- | --- |
| | | | |
| | | | |
| | | | |
| | | | |
| | | | |
| | | | |
| | | | |
| | | | |
| | | | |
| | | | |
| | | | |
| | | | |
| | | | |

## ADVANCED HEALTH RECORD

*Coding Clinic* and coding guidelines must be reviewed when coding records relating to poisoning, adverse effects of drugs, and injuries. A situation in which medication was taken incorrectly and not as it was prescribed will be considered a poisoning, whether or not the intent was to inflict harm. A situation in which the medication was taken as prescribed and the patient suffered harm would be considered an adverse effect. The QHCP will determine whether the medication was taken as prescribed.

The patient who attempts suicide and subsequently seeks medical attention is often seen in the ED, where measures are taken to reverse the effects of the ingested medication. At times, the overdose of a medication can create instability of the heart rhythm, kidney impairment, and stomach problems. The coder needs to add these secondary diagnoses to the coding abstract. The V code of suicidal ideation is applied in cases when a patient has indicated thoughts of suicide but has not actually made an attempt.

Based on the provided inpatient setting documentation, please assign the following:

- MS-DRG assignment
- ICD-9-CM diagnosis and procedure codes (FY2010)
- POA indicators

*ICD-9-CM and POA Coding Mentor,* edited by Patricia L. Bower-Jernigan, RHIA.

| | MS-DRG Assignment | | |
|---|---|---|---|

| ICD-9-CM Diagnosis Codes | ICD-9-CM Diagnosis Description | POA | Coding Clinic Reference/Reason |
|---|---|---|---|
| | | | |
| | | | |
| | | | |
| | | | |
| | | | |
| | | | |
| | | | |
| | | | |
| | | | |
| | | | |
| | | | |
| | | | |
| | | | |

| ICD-9-CM Procedure Codes | ICD-9-CM Procedure Description |
|---|---|
| | |
| | |
| | |
| | |
| | |

# Burns

## BASIC HEALTH RECORD

When reviewing a record of a patient with current burns of the body, the coder must look for several details in order to assign proper codes.

Burns are classified by degree. First-degree burns are described as superficial. They involve the top layer of the skin and are described as erythema, or redness of the skin. A first-degree burn may be swollen at the site and is painful to the patient.

Second-degree burns extend to the middle layer of skin, called the dermis. Blistering is often noted, weeping of the skin is seen, and the patient experiences pain.

Third-degree burns extend through all three layers of the skin and possibly deeper into internal structures. Because of the depth of these burns, patients lose their sweat glands, hair follicles, and nerve endings. Pain is not associated with a third-degree burn because of the loss of the nerve endings. However, third-degree burns are the most severe and have long periods of recovery and lasting impact on the patient.

In addition to the degree of burn, the coder needs to look for the extent of the burn. The QHCP should describe the burn area by a percentage of surface affected.

Finally, a cause for the burn must be described in the health record so that it may be captured in the coding abstract with an E code. If more than one external burn is documented in the record, the coder should sequence the highest-degree burn first, followed by the other listed burns. Review of coding guidelines and *Coding Clinic* on how to code burns is recommended.

Based on the provided inpatient setting documentation, please assign the following:

- MS-DRG assignment
- ICD-9-CM diagnosis codes (FY2010)
- POA indicators

## MS-DRG Assignment

| ICD-9-CM Diagnosis Codes | ICD-9-CM Diagnosis Description | POA | Coding Clinic Reference/Reason |
|---|---|---|---|
| | | | |
| | | | |
| | | | |
| | | | |
| | | | |

*ICD-9-CM and POA Coding Mentor,* edited by Patricia L. Bower-Jernigan, RHIA.
Copyright ©2010 Health Forum, Inc., an American Hospital Association company. All rights reserved.

# INTERMEDIATE HEALTH RECORD

Patients with extensive burns, as in the case of a third-degree burn, may require debridement of the affected area. This procedure may be an excisional debridement, which involves the use of a sharp instrument to remove more than loose fragments of tissue and is deep enough so that viable tissue is exposed, or a non-excisional debridement, which is performed through whirlpool baths, dressing changes, and wiping away of slough.

It is important for the coder to understand the difference between an excisional and a non-excisional debridement because coding guidelines and *Coding Clinic* indicate certain verbiage must be present in the health record in order to apply an excisional debridement code. This insight will guide the coder to know when further clarification is needed. If, for example, the QHCP does not identify the type of debridement as excisional or excised but the documentation indicates that this may be the type of debridement performed, the coder should generate a query asking for clarification. Appendix C provides guidelines and examples on how to write a query.

Based on the provided inpatient setting documentation, please assign the following:

- MS-DRG assignment
- ICD-9-CM diagnosis and procedure codes (FY2010)
- POA indicators

| | MS-DRG Assignment | | |
|---|---|---|---|

| ICD-9-CM Diagnosis Codes | ICD-9-CM Diagnosis Description | POA | Coding Clinic Reference/Reason |
|---|---|---|---|
| | | | |
| | | | |
| | | | |
| | | | |
| | | | |

| ICD-9-CM Procedure Codes | ICD-9-CM Procedure Description |
|---|---|
| | |
| | |
| | |
| | |
| | |

## ADVANCED HEALTH RECORD

Patients who present with burns need to be observed closely by the QHCP for secondary conditions that can arise. Electrolyte imbalances, fluid depletion, fluid overload, pain, nausea, and vomiting are all frequently observed and require attention with burn patients.

All documented secondary diagnoses need to meet one of the five criteria for reporting additional diagnoses as outlined in the general coding guidelines on reporting additional diagnoses: (1) clinical evaluation, (2) therapeutic treatment, (3) diagnostic procedures, (4) extended length of hospital stay, and (5) increased nursing care and/or monitoring. Each criteria should be considered for each secondary diagnosis. If one or more of these criteria are met, then the secondary diagnosis should be coded. However, if none of these five criteria is met, the secondary diagnosis listed in the health record should be excluded from the coding.

Based on the provided inpatient setting documentation, please assign the following:

* MS-DRG assignment
* ICD-9-CM diagnosis codes (FY2010)
* POA indicators

| | MS-DRG Assignment | | |
|---|---|---|---|
| | | | |

| ICD-9-CM Diagnosis Codes | ICD-9-CM Diagnosis Description | POA | Coding Clinic Reference/Reason |
|---|---|---|---|
| | | | |
| | | | |
| | | | |
| | | | |
| | | | |
| | | | |
| | | | |
| | | | |
| | | | |
| | | | |

# Factors Influencing Health Status and Other Contacts with Health Services

## BASIC HEALTH RECORD

Sudden onset of weakness, especially in the elderly, can be an alarming symptom of a greater problem. The extreme change from baseline activities and abilities is a helpful clinical indicator for the QHCP. This information can come from the patient, the caregiver, or family members much of the time.

When this symptom is reported, the QHCP begins the process of finding the underlying cause. If the symptom is accompanied by other symptoms, the QHCP may have a better idea of the underlying cause. After reviewing the diagnostic testing and lab results and considering the treatment regimen, if all the tests show levels within normal limits and the patient returns to his or her normal state of activity or ability, it may be necessary to apply a symptom code as the principal diagnosis.

If the coder suspects that clinical indicators may be present in the health record of a more specified diagnosis that was not documented by the QHCP, a query may be considered. See appendix C for assistance in writing a query.

Based on the provided inpatient setting documentation, please assign the following:

- MS-DRG assignment
- ICD-9-CM diagnosis codes (FY2010)
- POA indicators

| | MS-DRG Assignment | | |
|---|---|---|---|
| | | | |

| ICD-9-CM Diagnosis Codes | ICD-9-CM Diagnosis Description | POA | Coding Clinic Reference/Reason |
|---|---|---|---|
| | | | |
| | | | |
| | | | |
| | | | |
| | | | |

# INTERMEDIATE HEALTH RECORD

At times, a patient has a debilitating condition that prevents him or her from being discharged directly to home. If the patient meets criteria for acute and intensive rehabilitation services, he or she may be transferred to a unit that specializes in providing therapies directed at assisting the patient in regaining function with the goal of independence.

When coding the record of a patient who is admitted to undergo an acute rehabilitation process, the *Coding Clinic* and coding guidelines refer the coder to the use of a V code to be sequenced as the principal diagnosis. A code for the condition for which the patient is requiring rehabilitation should also be applied to the coding abstract.

Information within the coding guidelines and *Coding Clinic* also addresses the application of additional secondary codes. A procedure code for each specialized rehabilitation therapy should also be added to the coding abstract.

Based on the provided inpatient setting documentation, please assign the following:

- MS-DRG assignment
- ICD-9-CM diagnosis and procedure codes (FY2010)
- POA indicators

| MS-DRG Assignment |
| --- |
|  |

| ICD-9-CM Diagnosis Codes | ICD-9-CM Diagnosis Description | POA | Coding Clinic Reference/Reason |
| --- | --- | --- | --- |
|  |  |  |  |
|  |  |  |  |
|  |  |  |  |
|  |  |  |  |
|  |  |  |  |

| ICD-9-CM Procedure Codes | ICD-9-CM Procedure Description |
| --- | --- |
|  |  |
|  |  |
|  |  |
|  |  |
|  |  |

## ADVANCED HEALTH RECORD

Admission to an acute rehabilitation facility is necessary for some patients after surgery to help them to regain their preoperative functionality and to be able to return to independent living. Review of *Coding Clinic* and coding guidelines will assist the coder in accurate code selection for both the principal and secondary diagnoses.

The coder needs to carefully review the record to determine when and if it is appropriate to add codes for conditions still being documented that occurred during the acute hospital stay preceding the rehabilitation admission. All documented secondary diagnoses need to meet one of the five criteria for reporting additional diagnoses as outlined in the general coding guidelines on reporting additional diagnoses: (1) clinical evaluation, (2) therapeutic treatment, (3) diagnostic procedures, (4) extended length of hospital stay, and (5) increased nursing care and/or monitoring. Each criterion should be considered for each secondary diagnosis. If one or more of these criteria are met, then the secondary diagnosis should be coded. However, if none of these five criteria is met, the secondary diagnosis listed in the health record should be excluded from the coding.

Based on the provided inpatient setting documentation, please assign the following:

*   MS-DRG assignment
*   ICD-9-CM diagnosis and procedure codes (FY2010)
*   POA indicators

| MS-DRG Assignment | | | |
|---|---|---|---|

| ICD-9-CM Diagnosis Codes | ICD-9-CM Diagnosis Description | POA | Coding Clinic Reference/Reason |
|---|---|---|---|
| | | | |
| | | | |
| | | | |
| | | | |
| | | | |
| | | | |
| | | | |
| | | | |
| | | | |
| | | | |
| | | | |
| | | | |
| | | | |

| ICD-9-CM<br>Procedure Codes | ICD-9-CM Procedure Description |
|---|---|
|  |  |
|  |  |
|  |  |
|  |  |
|  |  |

# Multiple Significant Trauma

## BASIC HEALTH RECORD

Trauma victims who present to the hospital setting often will have sustained more than one injury. Determining the principal diagnosis for the coding abstract requires the coder to assess the noted injuries and the treatments associated with each. The injury that is most significant to the patient and has the majority of treatment surrounding it should be coded as the principal diagnosis. It is imperative that all other injuries also be assigned secondary codes.

Depending on the severity and number of injuries, the MS-DRGs assigned may be grouped in the MDC "multiple significant traumas." This MDC was created to account for situations in which more than one injury affects the patient. Final MDC and MS-DRG assignment should always be reviewed by the coder as a subsequent way to check the coding accuracy.

While contusions and fractures of the tissues and bones are painful and can require extensive treatment, injury to vital organs such as the heart, lungs, or kidneys may have a greater impact on the well-being of and final outcome for the patient. Always consider directly injured organs and the magnitude of the function they perform when determining the principal diagnosis.

Based on the provided inpatient setting documentation, please assign the following:

- MS-DRG assignment
- ICD-9-CM diagnosis and procedure codes (FY2010)
- POA indicators

*ICD-9-CM and POA Coding Mentor,* edited by Patricia L. Bower-Jernigan, RHIA.
Copyright ©2010 Health Forum, Inc., an American Hospital Association company. All rights reserved.

| MS-DRG Assignment |
|---|
|  |

| ICD-9-CM Diagnosis Codes | ICD-9-CM Diagnosis Description | POA | Coding Clinic Reference/Reason |
|---|---|---|---|
|  |  |  |  |
|  |  |  |  |
|  |  |  |  |
|  |  |  |  |
|  |  |  |  |
|  |  |  |  |
|  |  |  |  |
|  |  |  |  |
|  |  |  |  |
|  |  |  |  |

| ICD-9-CM Procedure Codes | ICD-9-CM Procedure Description |
|---|---|
|  |  |
|  |  |
|  |  |
|  |  |
|  |  |

# INTERMEDIATE HEALTH RECORD

Evaluation of the health record should always be conducted thoroughly by the coder to enable coding of each diagnosis to its greatest specificity. Fractures should be indicated in the health record as either closed or open.

A closed fracture—also called simple fracture—diagnosis indicates that an open wound did not result from the fracture. An open fracture—or compound fracture—diagnosis indicates that an open wound is present as a result of the fracture.

The coder should examine the record to determine what part of the bone is fractured. Specific codes both identify the part of the bone fractured and indicate whether the fracture is open or closed. In the case of multiple traumas, when assessing the record to determine which injury will be principal, the coder should assess the injuries that required surgical intervention. The diagnosis that requires the surgical intervention should be highly considered for the position of principal diagnosis.

Based on the provided inpatient setting documentation, please assign the following:

- MS-DRG assignment
- ICD-9-CM diagnosis and procedure codes (FY2010)
- POA indicators

| | MS-DRG Assignment | | |
|---|---|---|---|
| | | | |

| ICD-9-CM Diagnosis Codes | ICD-9-CM Diagnosis Description | POA | Coding Clinic Reference/Reason |
|---|---|---|---|
| | | | |
| | | | |
| | | | |
| | | | |
| | | | |
| | | | |
| | | | |
| | | | |
| | | | |
| | | | |
| | | | |
| | | | |
| | | | |

| ICD-9-CM Procedure Codes | ICD-9-CM Procedure Description |
|---|---|
| | |
| | |
| | |
| | |
| | |
| | |
| | |
| | |
| | |
| | |

# ADVANCED HEALTH RECORD

When preparing a coding abstract on a record that includes several co-morbidities and complications occurring during the stay, it is imperative that each diagnosis be captured to its greatest specificity through assignment of codes. The coding abstract should paint a portrait of the patient's current and overall health condition. This depiction reflects not only the actual diagnoses still present, for which the patient received monitoring, testing, and treatment, but also past diagnoses, which are captured through V codes.

Assigning procedure codes for surgical interventions as well as for diagnostic tests performed during the hospital stay is also important.

Based on the provided inpatient setting documentation, please assign the following:

- MS-DRG assignment
- ICD-9-CM diagnosis and procedure codes (FY2010)
- POA indicators

*ICD-9-CM and POA Coding Mentor,* edited by Patricia L. Bower-Jernigan, RHIA.
Copyright ©2010 Health Forum, Inc., an American Hospital Association company. All rights reserved.

**MS-DRG Assignment**

| ICD-9-CM Diagnosis Codes | ICD-9-CM Diagnosis Description | POA | Coding Clinic Reference/Reason |
|---|---|---|---|
| | | | |
| | | | |
| | | | |
| | | | |
| | | | |
| | | | |
| | | | |
| | | | |
| | | | |
| | | | |
| | | | |

*(Continued on next page)*

| ICD-9-CM Diagnosis Codes | ICD-9-CM Diagnosis Description | POA | Coding Clinic Reference/Reason |
|---|---|---|---|
|  |  |  |  |
|  |  |  |  |
|  |  |  |  |
|  |  |  |  |
|  |  |  |  |
|  |  |  |  |
|  |  |  |  |
|  |  |  |  |
|  |  |  |  |
|  |  |  |  |
|  |  |  |  |
|  |  |  |  |
|  |  |  |  |

| ICD-9-CM Procedure Codes | ICD-9-CM Procedure Description |
|---|---|
|  |  |
|  |  |
|  |  |
|  |  |
|  |  |
|  |  |
|  |  |
|  |  |
|  |  |
|  |  |

# Human Immunodeficiency Virus Infections

# BASIC HEALTH RECORD

Human immunodeficiency virus is a virus that can cause harm to the immune system. In its advanced stages, it is referred to as AIDS. Numerous coding guidelines and *Coding Clinic* are devoted to the HIV diagnosis. It is essential to review these in order to properly select the principal diagnosis and apply the correct HIV code. Additionally, the coder needs to determine whether the admission to the hospital is for an HIV-related condition; this determination will assist in choosing the correct principal diagnosis.

One of the requirements necessary to apply the HIV code is that the patient must have had an HIV-defining illness—one that resulted from the patient's positive HIV status. When the coder is unable to determine if the patient has had such a condition, it would be appropriate to query the QHCP. Review appendix C for guidelines on how to write a query.

As with any infectious process, review of the sepsis area of appendix A is helpful in determining if a query to the QHCP is appropriate.

Based on the provided inpatient setting documentation, please assign the following:

- MS-DRG assignment
- ICD-9-CM diagnosis codes (FY2010)
- POA indicators

| MS-DRG Assignment | | | |
| --- | --- | --- | --- |
| **ICD-9-CM Diagnosis Codes** | **ICD-9-CM Diagnosis Description** | **POA** | **Coding Clinic Reference/Reason** |
| | | | |
| | | | |
| | | | |
| | | | |
| | | | |
| | | | |
| | | | |
| | | | |
| | | | |
| | | | |

# INTERMEDIATE HEALTH RECORD

Whether a patient is newly diagnosed with HIV has no bearing on the sequencing of the principal diagnosis. The careful review of *Coding Clinic* and coding guidelines is highly recommended to gain an understanding of the most appropriate use of the HIV codes.

Once an HIV patient has been diagnosed with an HIV-related illness, he or she is to have a certain HIV code assigned to his or her coding abstracts from that time on. When it is not clear to the coder whether the patient has had any HIV-defining illnesses, it is appropriate to query the QHCP. See appendix C for assistance in formatting a query.

In any case of pneumonia that is not specified as to the type or the cause, it is recommended that the coder refer to the pneumonia section of appendix A as a guide to determining when to query for greater specificity. Likewise, in any case of an infectious process, it would be helpful for the coder to view the sepsis section of appendix A to determine whether any indication exists that a query would be suitable.

Based on the provided inpatient setting documentation, please assign the following:

- MS-DRG assignment
- ICD-9-CM diagnosis and procedure codes (FY2010)
- POA indicators

| MS-DRG Assignment |
|---|
|  |

| ICD-9-CM Diagnosis Codes | ICD-9-CM Diagnosis Description | POA | Coding Clinic Reference/Reason |
|---|---|---|---|
|  |  |  |  |
|  |  |  |  |
|  |  |  |  |
|  |  |  |  |
|  |  |  |  |
|  |  |  |  |
|  |  |  |  |
|  |  |  |  |
|  |  |  |  |
|  |  |  |  |

| ICD-9-CM Procedure Codes | ICD-9-CM Procedure Description |
|---|---|
|  |  |
|  |  |
|  |  |
|  |  |
|  |  |

# ADVANCED HEALTH RECORD

The QHCP may link the diagnosis of HIV to another diagnosis. When the coder follows the coding logic, two codes will be assigned to the coding abstract. Specific guidance is provided in *Coding Clinic* and coding guidelines regarding how to sequence HIV-related diagnoses. It is suggested that the coder review these.

When biopsies are conducted, it is helpful for the coder to look for the pathology report as it becomes available. If findings within that report provide insight into the disease process being experienced by the patient, it may be appropriate for the coder to query the QHCP for documentation of the results in the health record. A coder is not allowed to code the diagnosis that may be found within the pathology results. The diagnosis must be established by a QHCP in the health record. See appendix C for query formatting assistance.

Based on the provided inpatient setting documentation, please assign the following:

- MS-DRG assignment
- ICD-9-CM diagnosis and procedure codes (FY2010)
- POA indicators

| MS-DRG Assignment | | | |
|---|---|---|---|

| ICD-9-CM Diagnosis Codes | ICD-9-CM Diagnosis Description | POA | Coding Clinic Reference/Reason |
|---|---|---|---|
|  |  |  |  |
|  |  |  |  |
|  |  |  |  |
|  |  |  |  |
|  |  |  |  |
|  |  |  |  |
|  |  |  |  |
|  |  |  |  |
|  |  |  |  |
|  |  |  |  |
|  |  |  |  |
|  |  |  |  |
|  |  |  |  |
|  |  |  |  |
|  |  |  |  |

| ICD-9-CM Procedure Codes | ICD-9-CM Procedure Description |
|---|---|
|  |  |
|  |  |
|  |  |
|  |  |
|  |  |

| Query for QHCP |
|---|
|  |

*ICD-9-CM and POA Coding Mentor,* edited by Patricia L. Bower-Jernigan, RHIA.

# Clinical Workflow Process Tools

This appendix contains information that may be useful in situations where a specific diagnosis should be confirmed by the QHCP. It is important to review the clinical findings within the laboratory and radiology reports as well as the patient's described condition to determine if a more specific diagnosis can be established. It is equally important to look at the clinical findings for other common conditions often associated with that diagnosis. The use of this tool can help guide the coder to determine when a query may be appropriately initiated.

Please refer to the list of abbreviations in appendix D for help in interpreting any of the common abbreviations used in this appendix.

# ACUTE RESPIRATORY FAILURE

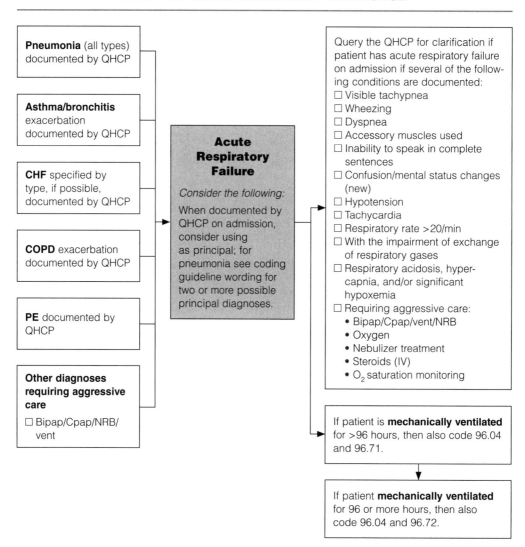

**Pneumonia** (all types) documented by QHCP

**Asthma/bronchitis** exacerbation documented by QHCP

**CHF** specified by type, if possible, documented by QHCP

**COPD** exacerbation documented by QHCP

**PE** documented by QHCP

**Other diagnoses requiring aggressive care**
☐ Bipap/Cpap/NRB/ vent

**Acute Respiratory Failure**

*Consider the following:*
When documented by QHCP on admission, consider using as principal; for pneumonia see coding guideline wording for two or more possible principal diagnoses.

Query the QHCP for clarification if patient has acute respiratory failure on admission if several of the following conditions are documented:
☐ Visible tachypnea
☐ Wheezing
☐ Dyspnea
☐ Accessory muscles used
☐ Inability to speak in complete sentences
☐ Confusion/mental status changes (new)
☐ Hypotension
☐ Tachycardia
☐ Respiratory rate >20/min
☐ With the impairment of exchange of respiratory gases
☐ Respiratory acidosis, hyper-capnia, and/or significant hypoxemia
☐ Requiring aggressive care:
  • Bipap/Cpap/vent/NRB
  • Oxygen
  • Nebulizer treatment
  • Steroids (IV)
  • $O_2$ saturation monitoring

If patient is **mechanically ventilated** for >96 hours, then also code 96.04 and 96.71.

If patient **mechanically ventilated** for 96 or more hours, then also code 96.04 and 96.72.

**References:**

• Per *Coding Clinic* 1st Quarter 2005, pages 7–8: If sepsis and acute respiratory failure both are present on admission, sepsis will be the principal diagnosis and acute respiratory failure will be the secondary diagnosis.

• Per *Coding Clinic* 3rd Quarter 2007, pages 7–8: If the patient has acute respiratory failure due to a poisoning, then the poisoning will be the principal diagnosis and acute respiratory failure will be the secondary diagnosis.

• Always refer to *Coding Clinic* for other specific examples of sequencing guidelines for respiratory failure.

# CHEST PAIN

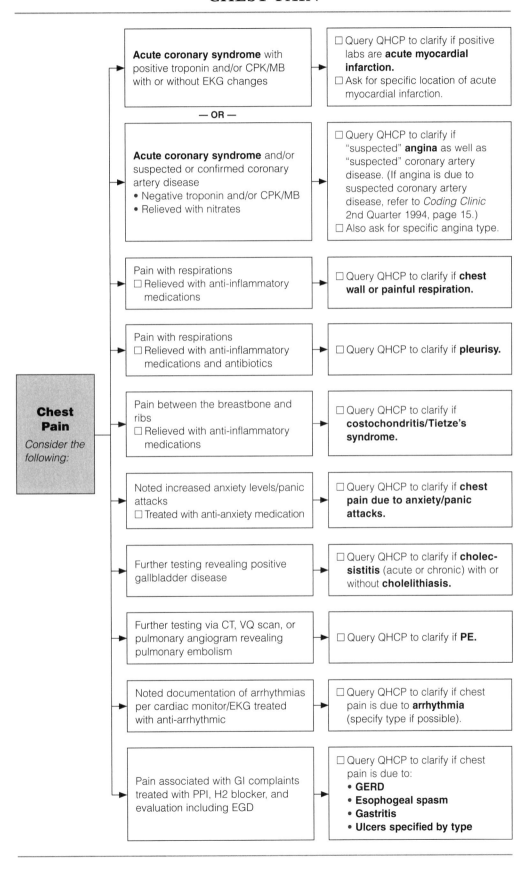

# CEREBRAL VASCULAR ACCIDENT

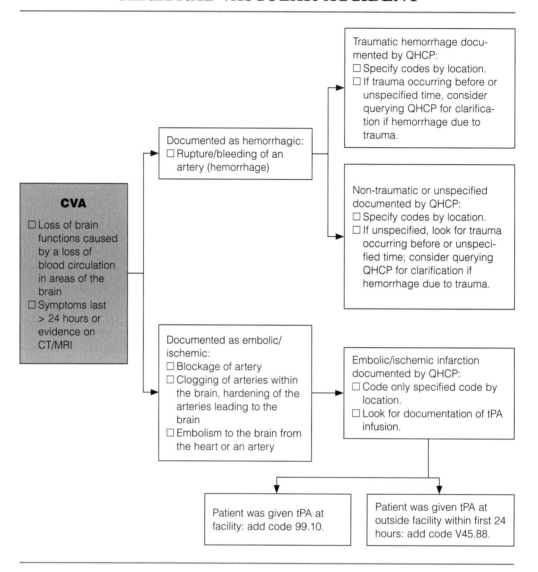

**CVA**

☐ Loss of brain functions caused by a loss of blood circulation in areas of the brain
☐ Symptoms last > 24 hours or evidence on CT/MRI

Documented as hemorrhagic:
☐ Rupture/bleeding of an artery (hemorrhage)

Traumatic hemorrhage documented by QHCP:
☐ Specify codes by location.
☐ If trauma occurring before or unspecified time, consider querying QHCP for clarification if hemorrhage due to trauma.

Non-traumatic or unspecified documented by QHCP:
☐ Specify codes by location.
☐ If unspecified, look for trauma occurring before or unspecified time; consider querying QHCP for clarification if hemorrhage due to trauma.

Documented as embolic/ischemic:
☐ Blockage of artery
☐ Clogging of arteries within the brain, hardening of the arteries leading to the brain
☐ Embolism to the brain from the heart or an artery

Embolic/ischemic infarction documented by QHCP:
☐ Code only specified code by location.
☐ Look for documentation of tPA infusion.

Patient was given tPA at facility: add code 99.10.

Patient was given tPA at outside facility within first 24 hours: add code V45.88.

# DIZZINESS

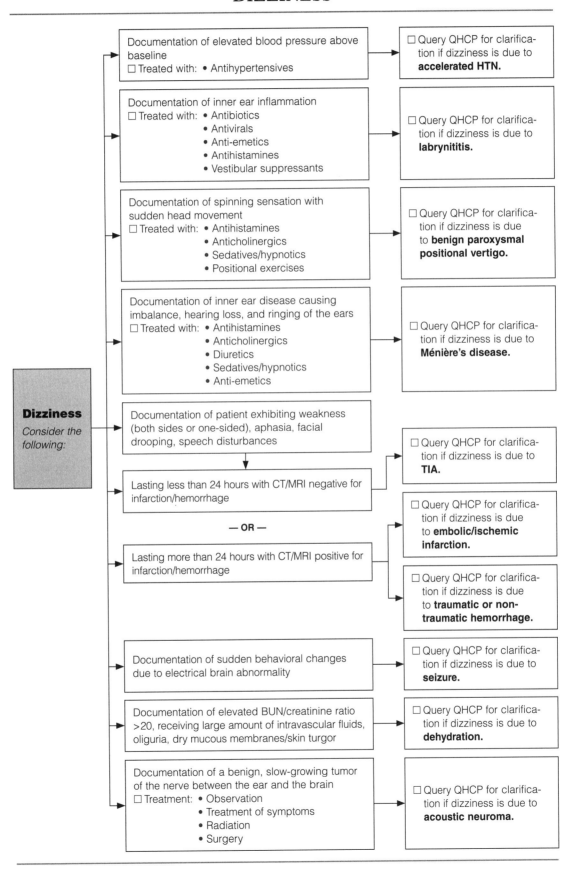

# PNEUMONIA

**Pneumonia**

*Consider the following:*

An inflammation of the lung, usually caused by an infection.
☐ Positive x-ray findings (remember that dehydrated patients on admit may not have a positive x-ray until they are rehydrated). Look for repeat x-ray findings and prompt for present on admission if not clarified by QHCP.
☐ Treated with antibiotics

---

Was patient noted to have:
☐ Dysphagia/evaluation of swallowing?
☐ Aspiration?
☐ History or current vomiting?
☐ Choking or gagging episodes?
☐ Recent or current seizures?
☐ Intoxication?
☐ Debilitation?
☐ Neurological impairment?

Treated with cefotetan, Unasyn, clindamycin, ampicillin, or imipenem, Zosyn, Timentin

→ ☐ Specify selected codes by what was aspirated.
☐ Query QHCP for clarification if **aspiration pneumonia.**

---

Was patient noted to have:
☐ Hospital acquired, institutional acquired, nursing home acquired?
Is patient:
☐ Compromised (immunosuppressed, long-term respiratory conditions, neurological impairment, cancer patient, organ transplant patient)?
☐ Common types confirmed if noted on sputum cultures (i.e., staphylococcal, gram negative *(Klebsiella, Pseudomonas, Enterobacter, Proteus, Serratia)*
☐ Treatment for gram negative: ceftazidime, Levaquin, cefepime, Fortaz, Timentin, Zosyn, gentamicin, aztreonam
☐ Treatment for *Staph aureus*: nafcillin, vancomycin

→ ☐ Query QHCP for clarification of type of pneumonia (organism) being treated for ("suspected" if not confirmed by cultures) but treatment supports **complex pneumonia.**

---

Is pneumonia noted to be:
☐ *Streptococcus*?
☐ *Haemophilus influenzae*?
☐ *Legionella*?
☐ *Mycoplasma*?
☐ *Chlamydia*?
☐ Virus?
☐ Simple/unspecified?

→ ☐ Query QHCP for clarification of type of pneumonia (organism) being treated (identified by culture results).

---

Was patient intubated with mechanical ventilation within the past 48 hours?
☐ Recent surgery requiring intubation/mechanical ventilation
☐ Short-term hospital stay with intubation/mechanical ventilation

→ ☐ Query QHCP for clarification if **ventilator-associated pneumonia.**

---

Does patient have **SIRS?**
☐ Fever
☐ Tachycardia
☐ Tachypnea
☐ Leukocytosis

---

Does patient have:
☐ Impairment of exchange of respiratory gases requiring aggressive care?
☐ Query the QHCP for clarification if patient has acute respiratory failure on admission if several of following conditions are documented:
☐ Visible tachypnea
☐ Wheezing
☐ Dyspnea
☐ Accessory muscles used
☐ Inability to speak in complete sentences
☐ Confusion/mental status changes (new)
☐ Hypotension
☐ Tachycardia
☐ Respiratory rate >20 min
☐ With the impairment of exchange of respiratory gases
☐ Respiratory acidosis, hypercapnia, and/or significant hypoxemia
☐ Requiring aggressive care:
  • Bipap/Cpap/vent/NRB
  • Oxygen
  • Nebulizer treatment
  • Steroids (IV)
  • O$_2$ saturation monitoring

→ ☐ If QHCP has documented sepsis and/or acute respiratory failure, and both were present on admission, apply coding guideline of two or more diagnoses that equally meet the definition for principal diagnosis, and select the most appropriate principal diagnosis (usually sepsis).

# RENAL FAILURE/DEHYDRATION

**Renal Failure/ Dehydration**

(abnormal BUN and creatinine lab values)

*Consider the following:*

---

Documentation of:
☐ Elevated BUN/creatinine ratio >20
☐ Receiving large amount of intravascular fluids
☐ Oliguria
☐ Dry mucous membranes/skin turgor

→ ☐ Query QHCP for clarification if patient has **dehydration.**

---

Documentation of:
☐ Hyperkalemia
☐ Acidosis
☐ Oliguria
☐ Dry mucous membranes/skin turgor
☐ Weakness/lethargy
☐ Tachycardia
☐ PLUS dramatic increase in BUN and creatinine levels from patient's baseline
☐ Focus of care on improving renal function

→ ☐ Query QHCP for clarification if patient has **acute renal failure.**
☐ Look for specific cause of acute renal failure:
  • Lupus nephritis
  • Hypertension
  • Due to diabetes mellitus
  • Postoperative (ex ATN; contrast induced, occurring with acute blood-loss anemia)
  • Post-traumatic
  • Renal cortical necrosis
  • Renal medullary necrosis
  • Tubular necrosis
☐ If known chronic kidney disease, refer to staging listed below.

---

Documentation of known chronic kidney disease with:
☐ GFR >90
☐ Creatinine >0.9

→ ☐ Query QHCP for clarification if patient has **stage I chronic kidney disease.**
☐ If on chronic dialysis, see end-stage renal disease.
☐ Look for specific cause of chronic renal failure.

---

Documentation of known chronic kidney disease with:
☐ GFR 60–89
☐ Creatinine 1.0–1.3

→ ☐ Query QHCP for clarification if patient has **stage II chronic kidney disease.**
☐ If on chronic dialysis, see end-stage renal disease.
☐ Look for specific cause of chronic renal failure.

---

Documentation of known chronic kidney disease with:
☐ GFR 30–59
☐ Creatinine 1.4–2.5

→ ☐ Query QHCP for clarification if patient has **stage III chronic kidney disease.**
☐ If on chronic dialysis, see end-stage renal disease.
☐ Look for specific cause of chronic renal failure.

---

Documentation of known chronic kidney disease with:
☐ GFR 15–29
☐ Creatinine 2.5–4.5

→ ☐ Query QHCP for clarification if patient has **stage IV chronic kidney disease.**
☐ If on chronic dialysis, see end-stage renal disease.
☐ Look for specific cause of chronic renal failure.

---

Documentation of known chronic kidney disease with:
☐ GFR <15
☐ Creatinine >4.5

→ ☐ Query QHCP for clarification if patient has **stage V chronic kidney disease.**
☐ If on chronic dialysis, see end-stage renal disease.
☐ Look for specific cause of chronic renal failure.

---

Documentation of known end-stage renal failure/disease (or) any stage chronic kidney disease requiring chronic dialysis

→ **End-stage renal failure/disease** documented by QHCP:
☐ If on chronic dialysis, see end-stage renal disease.
☐ Look for specific cause of **chronic renal failure.**

---

**Reference:**

GFR = glomerular filtration rate.

# SEPSIS

Respiratory infections documented:
☐ Pneumonia (all types)
☐ Bronchitis
☐ Other infections of respiratory tract

Nervous system infections documented:
☐ Meningitis (all types)
☐ Abscesses (all types)
☐ Encephalitis (all types)
☐ Myelitis (all types)
☐ Other infections of nervous system

Circulatory system infections documented:
☐ Endocarditis (all types)
☐ Pericarditis (all types)
☐ Myocarditis (all types)
☐ Other infections of circulatory system

Hepatobiliary system infections documented:
☐ Abscesses
☐ Other infections of hepatobiliary system

Kidney and urinary tract infections documented:
☐ UTI
☐ Pyelonephritis
☐ Urosepsis
☐ Other infections of kidney/urinary tract

Digestive system infections documented:
☐ Peritonitis
☐ Ruptured bowel with late presentation
☐ Ruptured appendicitis with late presentation
☐ *Clostridium difficile*
☐ Other infections of bowel/GI tract

Skin and subcutaneous tissue infections documented:
☐ Cellulitis
☐ Skin ulcerations (all types)
☐ Other infections of the skin/subcutaneous tissue

**Sepsis**

*Consider the following:*

When documented by QHCP on admission, consider using as co-principal rule. Consider querying QHCP for clarification if patient also has sepsis if several of following conditions are documented:
☐ New onset of mental changes that improve with antibiotic therapy
☐ Acidosis (pH < .32; $HCO_2$ <19 Hypotension
☐ Elevated temp >38.3°C or >101°F or diminished temp <36°C or 96.8°F.
☐ Greater than 90/min heart rate
☐ Greater than 20/min respiratory rate
☐ $PCO_2$
☐ Elevated WBC (12,000) or decreased WBC (4,000)
☐ Infection noted
☐ Treatment given for infection

Look for severe sepsis with end organ damage:
☐ QHCP must document link between organ damage involvement and sepsis in order to code.
☐ Types
• Acute respiratory failure
• Myopathy/polyneuropathy (critical illness)
• DIC
• Encephalopathy
• Hepatic failure
• Septic shock
• Acute renal failure
• Specify other types
☐ Consider querying QHCP to make linkage to sepsis.
☐ Add 995.92 in addition to specific codes for end organ damage diagnoses.

If patient **mechanically ventilated** for >96 hours, then also code 96.04 and 96.71.

If patient **mechanically ventilated** for 96 or more hours, then also code 96.04 and 96.72.

**Other noted infections to consider:**

| Postoperative infections | QHCP notes as postoperative infection. | Add 998.59 plus specified infection. |
| Infection due to device | QHCP links infection due to specified device. | Add specified codes by what device causing infection. |
| Infection with HIV | QHCP notes infection and HIV. | Add 042 plus specified infection. |

# SYNCOPE

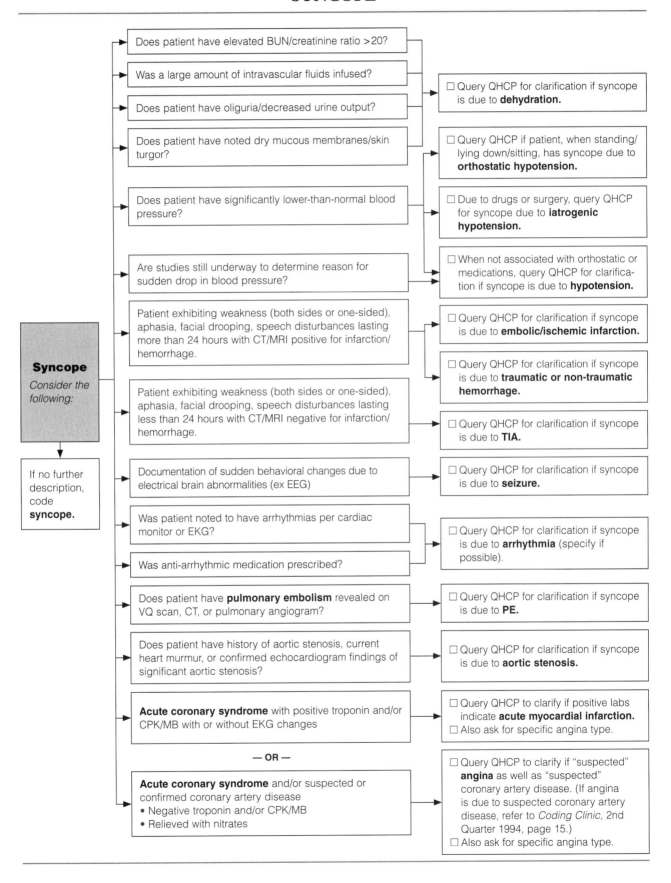

# URINARY TRACT INFECTION

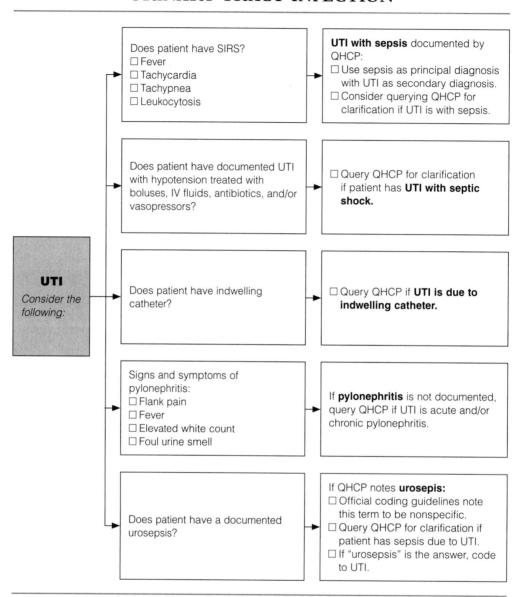

# Common Diagnosis Resource Indicators

This appendix is a reference the coder may consult for detailed descriptions of high-volume diagnoses. The appendix provides definitions and specific requirements of diagnoses, as well as the common clinical indicators that are seen with each of these diagnoses. This appendix will assist the coder in understanding the necessary clinical components when formulating a query, thus enabling him or her to achieve the greatest specificity of a diagnosis.

Please refer to the list of abbreviations in appendix D for help in interpreting any of the common abbreviations used in this appendix.

# ACUTE MYOCARDIAL INFARCTION

## Definitions

### Myocardial Infarction

An MI is characterized by the death of heart muscle cells due to abrupt loss of blood flow to a branch of a coronary artery.

#### Common Signs/Symptoms

Typical signs and/or symptoms of an MI include the following:

- Change in normal blood pressure (HTN or hypotension)
- Dyspnea
- Heavy, squeezing pressure; burning, crushing feeling
- Nausea and/or vomiting
- Paleness
- Palpitations
- Radiation of sensation to arms, abdomen, back, jaw, or neck
- Sweating
- Weakness

*Note:* Diabetic and elderly patients are more likely to present with atypical complaints (such as dyspnea, lightheadedness, nausea, and weakness) than are other types of patients.

Clinical findings that indicate MI include the following:

- A rise in troponin I is seen within four to six hours of the onset of MI and peaks between the second and fifth day, returning to normal by the seventh day. Any positive value indicates some injury. The troponin test shows a value of at least 0.6 and changes (increase/decrease) between troponin values.

*Note:* The troponin I test is the preferred lab study for diagnosing MI. Atrial fibrillation, CHF, bowel infarction, and renal failure may elevate troponins, so look for a change in these values.

- CPK rises within four to twenty-four hours (peaking at eighteen to twenty-four hours) and generally returns to normal by forty-eight to seventy-two hours.

*Note:* CPK totals may also rise due to muscular injections, CVAs, muscular diseases, trauma, and surgery. Small MIs may be missed by CPKs. Troponins are more useful indicators with these patients.

- LDH rises twenty-four to forty-eight hours after the occurrence of MI and remains elevated for seven to fourteen days.

### Risk Factors

Risk factors related to MI include the following:

- Connective tissue disease
- Diabetes mellitus
- Family history of CAD
- Hypercholesterolemia/hyperlipidemia
- HTN
- Increased age
- Inherited metabolic disorders
- Male
- Methamphetamine use
- Prior CVA
- Smoking history
- Stressful lifestyle

## Acute Coronary Syndrome

Typically, ACS is the initial diagnosis in AMI cases and is based entirely on history; risk factors; and, to a lesser extent, ECG findings. The symptoms arise from myocardial ischemia, the underlying cause of which is an imbalance between supply and demand of myocardial oxygen.

Patients with ACS include those whose clinical presentations cover the following range of diagnoses: unstable angina, NSTEMI, and STEMI.

*Note:* This ACS spectrum concept is a useful framework for developing therapeutic strategies but can often result in the AMI being missed in the documentation by the coder and thus alter the DRG assignment. It is important with ACS patients to consider the criteria to determine whether a query to the QHCP for an AMI is warranted.

## Angina

Angina symptoms result from myocardial oxygen insufficiency that can be the result of coronary disease (including spasm or syndrome X) or increased muscle mass. *Angina at rest* lasts less than ten minutes. *Accelerated angina pectoris* is an acute increase in symptoms, usually lasting more than ten minutes, that requires urgent diagnostic assessment.

*Note:* Once cardiac enzymes are substantially elevated, angina pectoris has evolved into an AMI.

### New York Heart Association Classification

*Class I:* Cardiac disease but without resulting limitation of activity. Does not cause undue fatigue, palpitation, dyspnea, or anginal pain. No objective evidence of cardiovascular disease.

*Class II:* Slight limitation of physical activity. Comfortable at rest. Ordinary physical activity results in fatigue, palpitation, dyspnea, or anginal pain. Minimal objective evidence of cardiovascular disease.

*Class III:* Marked limitation of physical activity. Comfortable at rest. Less than ordinary activity causes fatigue, palpitation, dyspnea, or anginal pain. Moderately severe objective evidence for cardiovascular disease.

*Class IV:* Inability to carry on any physical activity without discomfort. Symptoms of heart failure or anginal syndrome may be present even at rest. If any physical activity is taken on, discomfort is increased. Severe objective evidence for cardiovascular disease.

## Unstable Angina

Unstable angina occurs at rest and lasts for more than twenty minutes or is severe and started within the past month *or* is described as "crescendo pattern."

*Note:* Crescendo angina is a complication/co-morbidity.

## Chest Pain

Chest pain is not a diagnosis but rather is a symptom. As appropriate, look for or query the QHCP for further explanation of type and probable cause.

### *Type*

- Angina
- Biliary colic
- Heartburn
- Pleuritic/chest wall
- Radicular

### *Probable Cause*

- Angina
- Cocaine induced
- Costochondritis
- Gallstones
- GERD
- Musculoskeletal
- Pleurisy

# Difference between Angina and Non-anginal Pain

The differences between angina and non-anginal pain symptoms are detailed below.

## *Angina*

- Abates when stressor is gone or NTG is taken
- Lasts three to fifteen minutes
- Includes radiation to shoulder, neck, jaw, inner arm, epigastrium (can occur without chest component)
- Is relatively predictable
- Includes sensations in the chest of vise-like squeezing, heaviness, pressure, weight, aching, burning tightness

## *Non-anginal*

- Involves chest wall, is positional, is tender to palpations, can be infra-mammary; radiation patterns are highly variable
- Lasts seconds, minutes, hours, or all day
- Is pleuritic, sharp, pricking, knife-like, pulsating, choking
- Is characterized by random onset
- Responds to nitroglycerin variably

*Note:* If the QHCP documents "recent MI" in the patient's health record, clarify the time frame with the QHCP. Occurrence of the MI within eight weeks will still be considered acute for purposes of coding if it is the initial episode of care.

# CEREBRAL VASCULAR ACCIDENT

## Definitions

### CVA/Stroke

A CVA, also known as stroke, is the loss of brain functions caused by a loss of blood circulation to areas of the brain. A stroke is diagnosed if symptoms last more than twenty-four hours or evidence of CVA is found on a CT scan or an MRI.

#### Causes

The following are causes of a CVA:

- Blockage of artery (embolic/ischemic)
    —Clogging of arteries within the brain (for example, lacunar stroke)
    —Embolism to the brain from the heart or an artery
    —Hardening of the arteries leading to the brain (for example, carotid artery occlusion)
- Traumatic or non-traumatic rupture/bleeding of an artery (hemorrhage)
    —Cerebral hemorrhage (bleeding within the brain substance)
    —Ruptured aneurysm
    —Subarachnoid hemorrhage (bleeding between the brain and the inside of the skull)

### Transient Ischemic Attack

A TIA is characterized by transient neurological symptoms caused by ischemia lasting less than twenty-four hours and no evidence of a stroke on a CT scan or an MRI.

#### Causes

Causes of a TIA in patients include the following:

- Carotid stenosis
- Diffuse ASCVD
- Seizures

For coding purposes of a TIA, it is important that the physician specifically document the following in the health record:

- Acute or chronic
- Area of stroke
- Treatment patient received (tPA or interventions)
- Type of stroke (embolic or hemorrhage)

Note: If CVA is aborted, it is still appropriate to code the acute CVA if documented correctly. See *Coding Clinic* 1st Quarter 2007, pages 23–24.

# CONGESTIVE HEART FAILURE

# Definitions

## Congestive Heart Failure

Congestive heart failure is the inability of the heart to pump sufficient blood throughout the body.

## Acute CHF

Acute CHF is diagnosed based on the chest x-ray findings of pulmonary congestion or edema (conclusion often states "consistent with CHF"). Signs and symptoms of acute CHF include the following:

- Dyspnea
- Elevated BNP
- Orthopnea
- Paroxysmal nocturnal dyspnea
- Peripheral edema
- Shortness of breath

## Diastolic Congestive Heart Failure

Considered a "filling" problem, diastolic CHF is present when the left ventricle of the heart cannot relax or fill fully. Unable to relax between contractions (diastole), the heart cannot fill with sufficient blood because the heart muscle is stiff. Fluid builds up in the extremities first, but diastolic CHF can also lead to lung congestion. It is often a precursor to systolic congestive heart failure.

*Common signs* of diastolic CHF include lung congestion and lower extremity edema; ejection fracture remains at normal levels.

*Common causes* are HTN and cardiomyopathy.

## Systolic Congestive Heart Failure

Systolic CHF, a "pumping" problem, is diagnosed when the left ventricle of the heart cannot contract vigorously. It is unable to pump adequate amounts of blood during the contraction phase (systole). Blood coming from the lungs into the heart may back up and cause fluid leakage into the lungs, leading to pulmonary congestion.

*Common signs* of systolic CHF are lung congestion and lower extremity edema; ejection fracture levels are decreased.

*Common causes* are CAD, HTN or elevated BP, and valvular heart disease.

## Left-Sided Heart Failure

Left-sided heart failure is the inability of the heart's left ventricle to adequately pump oxygen-rich blood from the heart to the rest of the body.

*Common symptoms* of this type of heart failure are SOB, fatigue, cough, and orthopnea/PND.

*Common signs* are peripheral edema, elevated BNP, and an echocardiogram showing LVEF decreased to <50 percent.

*Common causes* are CAD, cardiomyopathy, stenosis, HTN, and valvular diseases.

## Right-Sided Heart Failure

Often referred to as cor pulmonale, in this condition, the heart's right ventricle does not have adequate ability to pump blood, causing fluid buildup in veins and swelling (edema). Right-sided heart failure is often seen with pulmonary disease patients because the right side of the heart cannot generate enough force to pump blood through a diseased lung.

*Common symptoms* of right-sided heart failure include chest pain on exertion, dyspnea, and SOB.

*Common signs* are edema and syncope and an echocardiogram showing decreased RVEF. The x-ray shows lung disease but no fluid (congestion), and often the patient has no history of CAD.

*Common causes* may be as a direct effect of left-sided heart failure, COPD, pulmonary disease, and pulmonary HTN.

## Treatment for CHF

The following treatment approaches and medications are indicated for CHF:

* *Low-sodium diet*

* *ACE inhibitors (brand names are shown in parentheses)*
  Benazepril (Lotensin)
  Captopril (Capoten)
  Enalapril (Vasotec)
  Fosinopril (Monopril)
  Lisinopril (Prinivil, Zestril)
  Moexipril (Univasc)
  Perindopril (Aceon)
  Quinapril (Accupril)
  Ramipril (Altace)
  Trandolapril (Mavik)

- *Beta-blockers  (brand names are shown in parentheses)*
  Acebutolol (Sectral)
  Atenolol (Tenormin)
  Betaxolol (Kerlone)
  Bisoprolol (Ziac)
  Bisoprolol/hydrochlorothiazide (Ziac)
  Careolol (Cartrol)
  Metoprolol (Lopressor, Toprol XL)
  Nadolol (Corgard)
  Propranolol (Inderal)
  Sotalol (Betapace)
  Timolol (Biocadren)

- *Calcium channel blockers (brand names are shown in parentheses)*
  Amlodipine (Norvasc, Lotrel)
  Bepridil (Vascor)
  Diltiazem (Cardizem, Tiazac)
  Felodipine (Plendil)
  Nifedipine (Adalat, Procardia)
  Nimodipine (Nimotop)
  Nisoldipine (Sular)
  Verapamil (Calan, Isoptin, Verelan)

- *Digitalis preparations*
  Digitoxin
  Digoxin
  Lanoxin

- *Diuretics (brand names are shown in parentheses)*
  Amiloride (Midamor)
  Bumetanide (Bumex)
  Chlorothiazide (Diuril)
  Chlorthalidone (Hygroton)
  Furosemide (Lasix)
  Hydrochlorothiazide (Esidrix, Dydrodiuril)
  Indapamide (Lozol)
  Spironolactone (Aldactone)

- *Dobutamine*

- *Dopamine*

- *Nitrates/vasodilators (brand names are shown in parentheses)*
  Hydralazine (Apresoline)
  Isosorbide dinitrate (Isordil)
  Minoxidil
  Nesiritide (Natrecor)
  Nitroglycerin (Nitro-Dur, Nitrolingual, Nitrostat, Transderm-Nitro, Nitropaste)

# MALNUTRITION

## Definitions

### Malnutrition

Malnutrition is defined as an imbalance between the body's needs and the person's intake of nutrients. This imbalance is most frequently associated with undernutrition, but it can also be attributed to overnutrition

#### Causes

The causes of malnutrition include the following:

- Conditions that decrease the body's ability to digest and absorb nutrients
  —Celiac disease
  —Cystic fibrosis
  —ETOH abuse
  —Malignancy
  —Pancreatic insufficiency
  —Pernicious anemia
  —Previous gastric bypass
  —Prolonged vomiting and diarrhea

- Conditions that lead to increased demand for nutrition
  —Infections
  —Malignancy
  —Ongoing wounds (surgical or chronic)
  —Severe burns
  —Surgery
  —Trauma
  —Uncontrolled or severe forms of diabetes

- Conditions that cause insufficient intake of nutrients
  —Chronic illness/conditions
  —Lack of ability to take in food (loss of appetite, poor dental health, swallowing ability, prolonged nausea)
  —Lack of food available (NPO, financial inability to obtain food)

- Conditions that lead to increased loss of nutrients
  —Chronic renal failure/chronic dialysis
  —Crohn's disease/inflammatory bowel disease
  —Diarrhea
  —Hemorrhaging
  —Vomiting

### Kwashiorkor

Kwashiorkor is a form of malnutrition caused by inadequate protein intake in the presence of fair to good energy (total calories) intake.

**Marasmus**

Marasmus is a severe form of malnutrition caused by inadequate intake of protein and calories. The condition usually occurs in the first year of life, resulting in wasting and growth retardation.

# Criteria for Malnutrition

Look for the following verbiage in the language used by the QHCP in the patient's health record:

- Cachexia
- Emaciated
- Frail
- Low BMI
- Malnutrition (to be staged)
- Thin
- Underweight

The patient type often seen with the following conditions are often diagnosed with malnutrition:

- Acute illnesses (severe)
- Alcoholism
- Chronic illness/disease
- Dementia/Alzheimer's disease/altered mentation
- Long hospitalization

The signs and symptoms of malnutrition are the following:

- Abnormal labs (total protein, albumin, pre-albumin, lipids, CBC, and metabolic panels)
- Anemia
- Brittle and malformed nails
- Chronic diarrhea
- Decreased immune response
- Decreased muscle mass
- Dizziness
- Dry, scaly skin
- Edema
- Fatigue/weakness
- Loss of hair pigment
- Mental changes (confusion/irritability)
- Slow-healing wounds
- Weight loss

*Note:* Most nutritionists would say that the pre-albumin is the most useful test in the acute setting for determining malnutrition.

# Treatment for Malnutrition

Paying attention to calorie counts; providing consultation with dietary experts; and providing supplemental feedings through TPN and/or feeding tubes are the main treatments for malnutrition.

Look for a combination of signs and symptoms and, especially, treatment directed toward malnutrition to determine whether to write a query to the QHCP.

Remember that patients *do not* need to be underweight to have malnutrition. Look at the patient's overall status to help decide if the QHCP should be queried for the diagnosis of malnutrition.

## Degrees of Malnutrition

Severe
      <70 percent IBW
      <16 BMI
      **Albumin <2.0**
      Transferrin <117
      **Prealbumin <5**
      Total lymphocyte count <900

Moderate
      70–79 percent IBW
      16–17 BMI
      **Albumin 2.1–2.9**
      Transferrin 117–133
      **Prealbumin 5–9**
      Total lymphocyte count 900–1,500

Mild
      80–89 percent IBW
      17–18.5 BMI
      **Albumin 3.0–3.4**
      Transferrin 134–175
      **Prealbumin 10–17**
      Total lymphocyte count 1,501–1,800

# PNEUMONIA

## Definitions

### Pneumonia

Pneumonia is an inflammation of the lung(s), usually caused by an infection. Three common causes are bacteria, viruses, and fungi. Pneumonia can also be caused by accidentally inhaling a liquid or chemical.

### Aspiration Pneumonia

Tiny particles from the mouth can slip or be inhaled (aspirated) into the airways. When such particles are not cleared by normal means (i.e., coughing), they can cause aspiration pneumonia. Older people and people who are debilitated, intoxicated by alcohol or drugs, or unconscious from anesthesia or a medical condition are especially at risk for this type of pneumonia, as are persons with impaired swallowing ability and those requiring tube feedings. Even a healthy person who inhales a large amount of material, as may happen during vomiting, can develop aspiration pneumonia.

### Community-Acquired Pneumonia

Community-acquired pneumonia is an infection or inflammation of the lungs that is generally acquired outside of a hospital or long-term care facility.

#### Common Types

Common types of community-acquired pneumonia include the following:

- *Chlamydia*
- *Haemophilus influenzae*
- *Legionella*
- *Mycoplasma*
- *Streptococcus*
- Viral

### Hospital-, SNF-, and Institution-Acquired Pneumonia

This designation of pneumonia is acquired in the hospital or another type of institution. It tends to be far more severe than pneumonia acquired in the community. The organisms in these institutions tend to be more aggressive, frequently are more resistant to antibiotics, and thus are harder to treat. People in hospitals and nursing homes tend to be sicker than those living in the community and therefore are not as able to fight the infection as easily.

### Common Types

Common types of pneumonia acquired in an institution are the following:

- Staphylococcal (complex pneumonia DRG)
- Gram negative (all complex pneumonia DRG)
- Actinomycosis
- *Enterobacter*
- *Klebsiella*
- *Proteus*
- *Pseudomonas*
- *Serratia*

## Ventilator-Associated Pneumonia

Ventilator-associated pneumonia is that which occurs in a person who has been assisted by mechanical ventilation within the past forty-eight hours. The QHCP must document the pneumonia as such; the coder must not assume the link between documentation and diagnosis.

# Signs and Symptoms of Pneumonia

## Simple and Complex

Both simple and complex cases of pneumonia can have the following symptoms:

- Cough (productive/dry)
- Dyspnea
- Fever
- Muscle pain
- Painful chest
- Possible confusion (especially with elderly)
- Shaking/chills/rigors
- Weakness

*Note:* The patient's health record must include positive x-ray findings during hospitalization (remember that a patient who is dehydrated upon admission may not test positive on x-ray until he or she is rehydrated). Look for repeat x-ray findings and prompt the QHCP for POA status if it is not clarified by the QHCP's documentation.

If sputum cultures test positive for a specified organism, query the QHCP to add the organism to the documentation

## Aspiration

Aspiration is indicated by the basic pneumonia criteria plus the following:

- Alcoholism
- Dementia, neurological illness/disorder that affects swallowing
- Documented choking, gagging spells, or abnormal swallow evaluation
- Emesis or witnessed aspiration
- Poor dentition
- Upper lobe infiltrates
- Treatment with cefotetan, clindamycin, Unasyn

## Complex Pneumonia Types

Complex pneumonia patient types are indicated by the basic criteria for pneumonia plus the following:

- Immuno-compromised
- Lung cancer (postobstructive infiltrate)
- Neurological illness (e.g., post-CVA, MS, ALS)
- Neutropenic
- Organ transplantation
- Recently hospitalized, or residing in another facility (nursing home, group home, multi-living environment)
- Severe COPD or lung disease
- Severely debilitated
- Tracheostomy or ventilator dependent

# Antibiotic Treatment for Pneumonia

Pneumonia that is diagnosed based on antibiotic treatment is characterized by the basic criteria for pneumonia *plus* the following:

- Gram negative (or possible, probable, suspected)—treatments include aztreonam, cefepime, ceftazidime (brand name Fortaz), gentamicin, Levaquin, Timentin, Zosyn
- *Staphylococcus aureus*—treatments include nafcillin, vancomycin

# Description of Pneumonia

Pneumonia that is diagnosed based on its description in addition to the basic criteria for pneumonia; is noted as hospital acquired, institution acquired, or SNF acquired; and falls under the more complex antibiotic treatment criteria, consider querying the QHCP for suspected type of organism.

*Note:* Also consider the criteria for acute respiratory failure and sepsis with these patient types.

# RESPIRATORY FAILURE

## Definitions

### Acute versus Chronic Respiratory Failure:

Acute hypercapnic respiratory failure develops over minutes to hours. As a result, the patient's pH level is significantly decreased, to lower than 7.3.

Chronic respiratory failure develops over several days or longer, allowing time for renal compensation and an increase in bicarbonate concentration. In this case, the patient's pH level is usually only slightly decreased.

*Note:* The distinction between acute and chronic hypoxemic respiratory failure cannot readily be made on the basis of arterial blood gas levels. The clinical data of chronic hypoxemia (such as polycythemia, severe COPD, or cor pulmonale) may help in suggestion of chronic respiratory failure.

### Acute Respiratory Distress

Acute respiratory distress is characterized by the following:

- Use of accessory muscles
- Cor pulmonale
- Confusion/mental status changes (new)
- Heart rate >100 bpm
- Hypotension (SBP <90, reduction from baseline by ≥40 mm Hg, or MAP <65)
- Inability to speak in complete sentences
- Respiratory rate >20 breaths/min
- Visible tachypnea/wheezing/dyspnea

*Note:* The lab test findings do not need to show an abnormality in the ABGs or the $O_2$ saturation monitoring for acute respiratory distress to be diagnosed.

### Acute Respiratory Failure

Acute respiratory failure is indicated by the following:

- Use of accessory muscles
- Confusion/mental status changes (new)
- Heart rate >100 beats/min
- Hypotension (SBP <90, reduction from baseline by ≥40 mm Hg, or MAP <65)
- Inability to speak in complete sentences
- Respiratory rate >20 breaths/min
- Visible tachypnea/wheezing/dyspnea

In combination with the impairment of exchange of respiratory gases, acute respiratory failure requires aggressive care and usually is manifested as a respiratory acidosis, hypercapnia, and/or significant hypoxemia.

*Note:* The patient does not have to be on a ventilator but should have frequent monitoring or respiratory treatments.

## When ABGs Are Normal

pH: 7.35–7.45 (critical values of <7.25 or >7.55)

$PaCO_2$: 35–45 mm Hg (critical values of <20 or >60 mm Hg)

$HCO_3$: 21–28 mEq/L (critical values of <15 or >40 mEq/L)

$PaO_2$: 80–100 mm Hg (critical values of <40 mm Hg)

$O_2$ saturation: 95–100 percent (critical values of 75 percent or lower)

## Hypercapnia

Hypercapnia is an increased amount of carbon dioxide in the blood caused by the body's inability to remove the carbon dioxide from it.

## Hypoxemia

Hypoxemia is insufficient oxygenation of blood caused by the body's inability to receive oxygen into it.

## Hypoxemic Respiratory Failure (type I)

Type I respiratory failure, hypoxemic, is characterized by a $PaO_2$ of less than 60 mm Hg with a normal or low $PaCO_2$. This is the most common form of respiratory failure, and it can be associated with virtually all acute diseases of the lung, which generally involve fluid filling or the collapse of alveolar units.

Some examples of type I respiratory failure are cardiogenic or non-cardiogenic pulmonary edema, pneumonia, sepsis, and pulmonary hemorrhage.

## Hypercapnic Respiratory Failure (type II):

Type II respiratory failure, hypercapnic, is characterized by a $PaCO_2$ of more than 50 mm Hg. Hypoxemia is common in patients with hypercapnic respiratory failure who are breathing room air. The pH level depends on the level of bicarbonate, which, in turn, is dependent on the duration of hypercapnia.

Common etiologies include drug overdose, neuromuscular disease, chest wall abnormalities, and severe airway disorders (e.g., asthma, COPD).

## SEPSIS

## Definitions

### Bacteremia

Bacteremia is bacteria in the blood without associated inflammatory response.

*Note:* This term is not to be interchanged with septicemia. Bacteremia denotes a laboratory finding, whereas septicemia denotes an acute illness. If SIRS is also present, querying the QHCP for clarification is recommended by *Coding Clinic.* When SIRS is present with positive blood cultures, consider querying for sepsis or septicemia.

### Sepsis

Sepsis is the systemic inflammatory response to a suspected or proven infection manifested by two or more of the SIRS conditions: fever, tachycardia, tachypnea, and leukocytosis. It is not the infection itself, but it is the result of or response to the infection.

### Septic Shock

Septic shock is sepsis with refractory hypotension where SBP <90 or MAP <65 and/or unresponsiveness to fluid resuscitation and hypoperfusion (lactic [metabolic] acidosis, oliguria, renal failure, hepatic failure, "altered mental status," myocardial or limb ischemia due to decreased BP or cardiac output).

### Septicemia

Septicemia is SIRS that is associated with the presence of pathological microorganisms or toxins in the blood, which can include bacteria, viruses, or fungi.

### Severe Sepsis

The severe form of sepsis is associated with organ failure with hypoperfusion (lactic [metabolic] acidosis, oliguria, renal failure, hepatic failure or shock liver, "altered mental status," myocardial or limb ischemia due to decreased BP or cardiac output) or hypotension.

### SIRS

This syndrome can be caused by suspected or known infection as well as non-infectious conditions (e.g., pancreatitis, burns, trauma).

### Urosepsis

Urosepsis is pyuria or bacteria in the urine (not in the blood).

*Note:* The term *urosepsis* is often used when SIRS is present along with infection of the urinary tract. Querying the QHCP for clarification of UTI with sepsis is recommended by *Coding Clinic.*

# Coding Sepsis

## Sepsis

### Strong Signs of Sepsis

Particularly strong signs that indicate sepsis include the following:

- Acidosis (pH <7.32, HCO$_3$ <19)
- Hypotension (SBP <90 mm Hg, MAP <65, or SBP <40 mm Hg of patient's baseline).
- New onset of mental changes that improve with antibiotic therapy (within seventy-two hours)

One of the three signs from the above list must be present for sepsis to be connected to pneumonia

### Other Signs of Sepsis (SIRS)

*Note:* Recently added criteria dictate that two or more of the following signs must be present to determine sepsis.

- Cardiac index >3.5 L/min/m$^2$ (not explained by other causes). It may be helpful to determine if the patient has undergone Swan-Ganz catheterization.
- Elevated temp >38.3°C or >101°F. Diminished temp <36°C or 96.8°F.
- Elevated WBC (12,000) or decreased WBC (4,000). If the WBC is normal and there is no left shift/bandemia (left shift: increase in neutrophils), it is very difficult to substantiate that the patient has sepsis.
- Greater than 20 breaths/min respiratory rate.
- Greater than 90 bpm heart rate.
- History of sepsis.
- Hyperglycemia (plasma glucose 120 mg/dl or greater) in absence of diabetes.
- Increase in neutrophils by >10 percent (left shift: increase in neutrophils, PMN bandemia 85 percent).
- Infectious focus.
- PCO$_2$ <32.
- Significant edema or positive fluid balance (20 ml/kg over twenty-four hours).
- Urine output <30 cc/hr
  —Oliguria/anuria (<0.5 cc/kg/hr for one hour despite fluid resuscitation).

Septicemia treatment includes the procedures mentioned above and positive blood cultures.

### Treatments

Treatments for sepsis may include the use of vasopressors (or "pressors") for severe sepsis/septicemia. Also applied are rapid rehydration (4 liters in <six hours) and IV antibiotics.

## Severe Sepsis

With severe sepsis, organ dysfunctions (not explained by other causes) are present. Coding for this condition requires documentation of organ damage; the QHCP MDs must make the link between sepsis and the following:

- Acute renal failure
- Acute respiratory failure
- DIC
- Encephalopathy
- Hepatic failure/liver failure/shock liver/liver infarction
- Myopathy/polyneuropathy (critical illness)
- Septic shock
- Specify other types

Blood dysfunction

- Acute anemia
- Increased APTT
- Elevated D-dimer
- Thrombocytopenia (<80,000, or 50 percent decrease over the past three days)
- Metabolic acidosis
  —lactic acidosis: pH <7.3 and plasma lactate >1.5 times normal

Cardiovascular dysfunction

- Hypotension
- Tachycardia

Gastrointestinal/endocrine dysfunction

- Acute GI bleed/acute pancreatitis
- Intestinal ischemia

Hepatic dysfunction

- Documentation of liver failure, shock liver, stunned liver, liver infarction
  —Decreased albumin and increased PT
  —Jaundice with elevated liver enzymes
- Neurological dysfunction
  —Acute encephalopathy
  —Alteration in consciousness/confusion/psychosis
- Renal dysfunction
  —Documentation of acute renal failure. When coding, look at the criteria to determine whether it meets the requirements for querying the QHCP.
- Respiratory dysfunction
  —Documentation of acute respiratory failure

## Pediatric SIRS

To diagnose pediatric SIRS, the QHCP needs to see at least two of the following present, and one of these must be abnormal temperature or leukocyte count.

- Core temperature of >38.5°C or <36°C
- Elevated or depressed WBC or >10 percent bands
- Increased respiratory rate
- Tachycardia
- No secondary causes for the above

# Qualified Health Care Professional Query Guidelines and Tools

This appendix contains information for a coder who, after review of the clinical findings within the laboratory and radiology reports as well as the patient's described condition, determines that a query to the QHCP is appropriate.

When creating a query, it is important that all pertinent data and treatment directed toward the condition be identified within the context of the query. The following introduction to the query process, reprinted from a practice brief published by the American Health Information Management Association (AHIMA), provides straightforward guidance for writing an effective query.

As stated by AHIMA:

> This practice brief offers HIM professionals important components to consider in the management of an effective query process. It is intended to offer guiding principles to implement the query process while in no way prescribing what must be done.

Please refer to the list of abbreviations in appendix D for help in interpreting any of the common abbreviations used in this appendix.

## AHIMA QUERY GUIDELINES

# A Query

A qualified health care provider should be queried for clarification and additional documentation prior to code assignment when there is conflicting, incomplete, or ambiguous information in the health record regarding a significant reportable condition or procedure or other reportable data element dependent on health record documentation.

## When Formatting the Query

- It is recommended to state the issue in the form of a question along with clinical indicators specified from the health record and asking the provider to make a clinical interpretation of these facts based on his or her professional judgment of the case.

- The query should not be designed to ask questions about a diagnosis or procedure that can be responded to in a yes/no fashion.

    —The exception is present on admission (POA) queries when the diagnosis has already been documented.

- Ask the provider to document the diagnosis he or she is agreeing to. Concerns about yes/no queries are less of an issue if the entity requires the provider to document the diagnosis in the health record rather than relying on the query form for the final documentation.

- Multiple choice formats that employ checkboxes may be used as long as all clinically reasonable choices are listed, regardless of the impact on reimbursement or quality reporting. The choices should also include an "other" option, with a line that allows the provider to add free text. Providers should also be given the choice of "unable to determine."

- A single query form can be used to address multiple questions. If it is, a distinct question should be asked for each issue (e.g., if three questions exist based on clinical indications in the health record, there should be three distinct questions clearly identified on the query form).

- Never indicate that a particular response would favorably or unfavorably affect reimbursement or quality reporting.

Source: American Health Information Management Association, *Managing an Effective Query Process* (AHIMA Practice Brief), *AHIMA Journal,* Oct. 2, 2008. Reprinted with permission of AHIMA. This practice brief offers HIM professionals important components to consider in the management of an effective query process. It is intended to offer guiding principles to implement the query process while in no way prescribing what must be done.

# CEREBRAL VASCULAR ACCIDENT

## Scenario

Patient admitted with confusion, right arm weakness, right facial droop upon awakening. Patient has known history of left carotid stenosis.

MRI results: acute infarct of left lacunar region

Lab work: sodium 124

## Admitting diagnosis

TIA versus CVA

Left carotid stenosis

Hyponatremia

## Other conditions noted in chart

Previous TIA, hyperlipidemia, past smoking history with mild COPD

## Hospital stay

Patient was evaluated in ED and determined that tPA was not appropriate due to unknown onset of symptoms. Patient was started on IV heparin infusion and IV fluids.

Patient was seen by physical and occupational therapy.

Patient's confusion cleared, but right arm weakness and right facial droop continued through hospital stay.

Documentation through stay altered between CVA and TIA. Patient was sent to transitional care facility for further physical and occupational therapy.

## Discharge diagnosis

TIA

CVA

Left carotid stenosis

Hyponatremia

## Query written for clarification of principal diagnosis

Dear QHCP:

Patient was admitted with confusion, right arm weakness, and right facial droop. MRI results indicated acute infarct of left lacunar region. Patient has known left carotid stenosis. Patient was discharged with continued right arm weakness and right facial droop. Discharge summary notes both TIA and CVA as diagnoses. Please clarify, after study, which diagnosis is considered to be principal diagnosis for this stay.

If CVA is determined to be the principal diagnosis, please further describe by acuity (acute, chronic) and location of the infarction.

Thank you.

# HEART FAILURE

## Scenario

Patient admitted with chest heaviness and shortness of breath.
- EKG: acute anterior myocardial infarction
- X-ray: acute pulmonary congestion consistent with heart failure
- Lab work: troponins 1.21, CPK 520, MB index of 23
- BNP: 953

## Admitting diagnosis

Acute anterior myocardial infarction
Heart failure

## Other conditions noted in chart

CAD, hyperlipidemia, morbid obesity with a BMI >40

## Hospital stay

Patient was taken immediately to the cardiovascular lab for an angiogram with a PTCA/drug-eluting stent placed. Echocardiogram results: systolic dysfunction with EF of 30%. IV Lasix given ×3 doses and placed on a daily oral Lasix.

Patient started on oral Vasotec and Lopressor.

Heart failure education and instructions given.

Patient was discharged three days later.

## Discharge diagnosis

Acute anterior myocardial infarction
Heart failure
CAD
Hyperlipidemia
Morbid obesity

## Query written for heart failure specifics

Dear QHCP:

Heart failure is documented on admission with BNP 953; noted shortness of breath with IV Lasix ×3 given; and started on oral Lasix, Vasotec, and Lopressor.

Echocardiogram results were systolic dysfunction with EF of 30%. For completeness of record, please consider further documentation of the type (diastolic, systolic, both, other) and the acuity (acute, chronic, both) of heart failure patient was treated for.

Thank you.

# MALNUTRITION

## Scenario

Patient is admitted with sharp abdominal pain with no bowel movement for five days.

Patient has known metastasic cancer of the liver and bone.

Patient has been decreasing in weight over past four months with limited appetite. Currently patient's BMI is 17.3.

Abdominal x-ray shows small-bowel obstruction.

Lab work: albumin 1.9, protein 4.7.

## Admitting diagnosis

Small-bowel obstruction
Metastasic cancer of liver
Metastasic cancer of bone

## Other conditions noted in chart

Underweight, depression

## Hospital stay

Patient was placed on a bowel rest program including IV fluids, nasogastric tube, and anti-emetics. Nutritionist was consulted and, per recommendation, patient had a PICC line placed and TPN and lipids were started. Pre-albumin lab: 4. After four-day stay, patient had bowel function, and QHCP ordered transitional care and continued TPN and lipid administration. Patient was transferred to transitional care facility.

## Discharge diagnosis

Small bowel obstruction
Metastasis cancer of liver
Metastasis cancer of bone
Underweight
Depression

## Query written for clarification of diagnosis under treatment

Dear QHCP:

Patient was started on TPN and lipids per recommendation of the nutritionist, with albumin 1.9, protein 4.7, and prealbumin 4. Patient is noted to have had decreasing weight with limited appetite past four months with noted diagnosis of underweight and BMI of 17.3. Please clarify if patient was started on TPN and lipids for any of the following:

- Severe malnutrition
- Moderate malnutrition
- Mild malnutrition
- Underweight
- Other
- Prophylactically administrated

Thank you.

# PNEUMONIA

## Scenario

Patient admitted with sudden SOB with weakness and chills.
Chest x-ray revealed RLL pneumonia.
Sputum cultures: *Streptococcus pneumoniae*
Lab work: WBC 18.3

## Admitting diagnosis

RLL pneumonia

## Other conditions noted in chart

CAD with past MIs with PTCA/stent and CABG, chronic systolic CHF/
ischemic cardiomyopathy, COPD with home $O_2$ dependency.

## Hospital stay

Patient treated with IV antibiotics ciprofloxacin and Zosyn, plus ongoing home
medications.

Patient was discharged after four days of IV antibiotic treatment with improved
respiratory symptoms. Sent home on oral antibiotics and continued home
medications/oxygen as before admission.

## Discharge diagnosis

RLL pneumonia
Chronic systolic CHF
CAD
Cardiomyopathy
COPD

## Query written for pneumonia specifications

Dear QHCP:

Patient was admitted with RLL pneumonia. Patient received IV ciprofloxacin
and IV Zosyn. Sputum cultures results showed *Streptococcus pneumoniae*. For
completeness of record, please clarify if a known or suspected type of pneumonia
was treated.

Thank you.

# RESPIRATORY FAILURE

## Scenario

Patient admitted with extreme shortness of breath, gasping breaths between words, respiratory rate 40 breaths/min, heart rate 130 bpm.
Chest x-ray reveals acute pulmonary congestion compatible with heart failure.
Lab work: BNP 1,400; ABGs pH 7.19; $PCO_2$ 65, $PO_2$ 40 with $O_2$ saturation 75% on room air

## Admitting diagnosis

Acute on chronic systolic heart failure

## Other conditions noted in chart

CAD, chronic kidney disease stage II, hypertension

## Hospital stay

Patient initially received IV Bumex and was placed on 80% facemask. The following day, patient was able to speak in full sentences and reduced to 2 liters per nasal cannula $O_2$. Patient had home diuretics and other heart failure medications adjusted through stay. Patient was discharged five days later.

## Discharge diagnosis

Acute on chronic systolic heart failure
CAD
Chronic kidney disease stage II
Hypertension

## Query written for clarification of complex respiratory treatment

Dear QHCP:

Upon admission to hospital, patient described as "gasping" with respiratory rate 40 breaths/min; HR 130 bpm; ABGs, pH 7.19, $PCO_2$ 65, $PO_2$ 40 with $O_2$ saturation 75% on room air. Patient was placed on 80% facemask with IV Bumex given. For completeness of record, please clarify if, in addition to the acute on chronic systolic heart failure, there are any specific respiratory diagnoses for patient (e.g., acute respiratory failure, acute respiratory distress, hypoxia, other).

Thank you.

# SEPSIS

## Scenario

Patient admitted with fever of 103°F, BP 80/42, HR 120, RR 30. Patient is confused to time, place. Patient is currently under outpatient treatment for left lower leg cellulitis with oral antibiotics.
Lab work: WBC 24,000

## Admitting diagnosis

Systemic illness due to infection
Left lower leg cellulitis
Confusion due to infection
Hypotension due to infection
Tachycardia due to infection

## Other conditions noted in chart

Chronic kidney disease stage II

## Hospital stay

Patient was admitted to ICU with central line placement, IV dopamine infusion, IV fluids @ 125 cc/hr, and IV vancomycin, and was treated by wound care specialist. Patient improved, with vital signs stabilizing, and patient became oriented within 36 hours of admission. Patient was transferred to medical floor after three days in ICU and was discharged two days later with ongoing home health care.

## Discharge diagnosis

Systemic illness due to infection
Left lower leg cellulitis
Confusion due to infection
Hypotension due to infection
Tachycardia due to infection
Chronic kidney disease stage II

## Query written for clarification of "systemic illness"

Dear QHCP:

"Systemic illness due to infection" is noted as a diagnosis with noted confusion, hypotension, tachycardia, and WBC 24,000.

Patient was treated with IV dopamine and IV vancomycin. Left lower leg cellulitis is noted as source of infection. Please clarify if any of the following would be appropriate to further define "systemic illness due to infection" noted in chart.
• SIRS due to cellulitis
• Sepsis due to cellulitis
• Septic shock due to cellulitis
• Other defined diagnosis _____
• No further description

Thank you.

# Common Abbreviations

This appendix is a reference to aid the coder in interpreting any of the common abbreviations used throughout the workbook and answer key. The list is in alphabetical order by abbreviation.

ABGs . . . . . . . . arterial blood gases

ACE . . . . . . . . . angiotensin-converting enzyme

ACS . . . . . . . . . acute coronary syndrome

AHIMA . . . . . . . American Health Information Management Association

AIDS . . . . . . . . acquired immunodeficiency syndrome

ALS. . . . . . . . . . amyotrophic lateral sclerosis

AMI. . . . . . . . . . acute myocardial infarction

APTT. . . . . . . . . activated partial thromboplastin time

ASA. . . . . . . . . . acetylsalicylic acid

ASCVD . . . . . . . atherosclerotic cerebral vascular disease

ATN. . . . . . . . . . acute tubular necrosis

AVR. . . . . . . . . . aortic valve replacement

BHP . . . . . . . . . benign hypertrophy of the prostate

Bipap . . . . . . . . bi-level positive airway pressure

BMI. . . . . . . . . . body mass index

BNP . . . . . . . . . brain natriuretic peptide

BP. . . . . . . . . . . blood pressure

BPH . . . . . . . . . benign prostate hypertrophy

bpm . . . . . . . . . beats per minute

BUN . . . . . . . . . blood urea nitrogen

C. . . . . . . . . . . . Celsius or centigrade

CABG . . . . . . . . coronary artery bypass graft

CAD . . . . . . . . . coronary artery disease

CAT. . . . . . . . . . computerized axial tomography

CBC . . . . . . . . . complete blood count

CC . . . . . . . . . . central catheter

cc/hr . . . . . . . . cubic centimeters per hour

cc/kg/hr. . . . . . . cubic centimeters per kilogram per hour

CHF . . . . . . . . . congestive heart failure

CKD . . . . . . . . . chronic kidney disease

COPD . . . . . . . . chronic obstructive pulmonary disease

Cpap. . . . . . . . . continuous positive airway pressure

CPB . . . . . . . . . cardiopulmonary bypass

CPK . . . . . . . . . creatine phosphokinase

CPT. . . . . . . . . . Current Procedural Terminology

CSF. . . . . . . . . . cerebrospinal fluid

CT. . . . . . . . . . . *see* CAT

CVA. . . . . . . . . . cerebral vascular accident

DIC . . . . . . . . . . disseminated intravascular coagulation

DKA . . . . . . . . . diabetic ketoacidosis

DRG . . . . . . . . . diagnosis-related group

DT. . . . . . . . . . . delirium tremens

E code . . . . . . . external cause of injury code

ECG . . . . . . . . . electrocardiogram

ECT. . . . . . . . . . electroconvulsive therapy

ED. . . . . . . . . . . emergency department

EEG . . . . . . . . . electroencephalography

EF. . . . . . . . . . . ejection fraction

EGD . . . . . . . . . esophagogastroduodenoscopy

EKG . . . . . . . . . *see* ECG

ESRD . . . . . . . . end-stage renal disease

ETOH . . . . . . . . ethanol

ex . . . . . . . . . . . example

F. . . . . . . . . . . . Fahrenheit

FY. . . . . . . . . . . fiscal year

GBS . . . . . . . . . group B *Streptococcus*

GERD . . . . . . . . gastroesophageal reflux disease

GFR . . . . . . . . . glomerular filtration rate

GI . . . . . . . . . . . gastrointestinal

H2. . . . . . . . . . . histamine H2-receptor

HCO$_3$ . . . . . . . . bicarbonate

Hct . . . . . . . . . . hematocrit

HCTZ . . . . . . . . hydrochlorothiazide

Hg . . . . . . . . . . . mercury

Hgb . . . . . . . . . . hemoglobin

HIM . . . . . . . . . . health information management

HIV . . . . . . . . . . human immunodeficiency virus

HR . . . . . . . . . . heart rate

HTN . . . . . . . . . hypertension

i.e. . . . . . . . . . . . that is

IBW . . . . . . . . . . ideal body weight

ICU . . . . . . . . . . intensive care unit

IFSE . . . . . . . . . internal fetal scalp electrode

IV . . . . . . . . . . . intravenous

kg/m$^2$ . . . . . . . . kilograms per meter squared

L/min/m$^2$ . . . . . . liters per minute per square meter

LDH . . . . . . . . . lactate dehydrogenase

LFT . . . . . . . . . . liver function test

LH . . . . . . . . . . . left handed

LVEF . . . . . . . . . left ventricular ejection fraction

MAP . . . . . . . . . mean arterial pressure

MB . . . . . . . . . . muscle band

MDC . . . . . . . . . Major Disease Category

mEq/L . . . . . . . . milliequivalents per liter

mg . . . . . . . . . . . milligram

mg/dl . . . . . . . . milligrams per deciliter

MI . . . . . . . . . . . myocardial infarction

min . . . . . . . . . . minute

ml/kg . . . . . . . . milliliters per kilogram

mm . . . . . . . . . . millimeters

MM . . . . . . . . . . multiple myeloma

MRI . . . . . . . . . . magnetic resonance imaging

MRSA . . . . . . . . methicillin-resistant *Staphylococcus aureus*

MS . . . . . . . . . . multiple sclerosis

MS-DRG . . . . . . Medicare severity diagnosis-related group

NPO . . . . . . . . . nothing per os (nothing per mouth)

NRB . . . . . . . . . non-rebreather (mask)

NSTEMI . . . . . . . non–ST-elevation myocardial infarction

NSVT . . . . . . . . . nonsustained ventricular tachycardia

NTG . . . . . . . . . nitroglycerin

$O_2$ . . . . . . . . . . . oxygen

$PaO_2$ . . . . . . . . partial pressure of oxygen

$PaCO_2$ . . . . . . . pressure of carbon dioxide

PE . . . . . . . . . . . pulmonary embolism

pH . . . . . . . . . . . power of hydrogen

PICC . . . . . . . . . peripherally inserted central catheter

PMN . . . . . . . . . polymorphonuclear neutrophils

PND . . . . . . . . . paroxysmal nocturnal dyspnea

POA . . . . . . . . . present on admission

PPI . . . . . . . . . . proton pump inhibitor

prn . . . . . . . . . . as needed

PT . . . . . . . . . . . prothrombin

PTCA . . . . . . . . . percutaneous transluminal coronary angioplasty

QHCP . . . . . . . . qualified health care provider

QT . . . . . . . . . . . Q wave and T wave intervals

RBC . . . . . . . . . red blood cell, red blood count

RLL . . . . . . . . . . right lower lobe

RR . . . . . . . . . . . respiratory rate

RVEF . . . . . . . . right ventricular ejection fracture

SAH . . . . . . . . . subarachnoid hemorrhage

SBO . . . . . . . . . small bowel obstruction

SBP . . . . . . . . . systolic blood pressure

SIADH . . . . . . . . syndrome of inappropriate antidiuretic hormone

SIRS . . . . . . . . systemic inflammatory response syndrome

SNF . . . . . . . . . skilled nursing facility

SOB . . . . . . . . short(ness) of breath

SSI . . . . . . . . . . sliding-scale insulin

STEMI . . . . . . . ST-elevation myocardial infarction

temp . . . . . . . . temperature

TIA . . . . . . . . . . transient ischemic attack

TNM . . . . . . . . tumor, node, metastasis

tPA . . . . . . . . . . tissue plasminogen activator

TPN . . . . . . . . . total parenteral nutrition

TURP . . . . . . . . transurethral resection of the prostate

UTI . . . . . . . . . . urinary tract infection

V code . . . . . . . screening code

vent . . . . . . . . . ventilator

VQ . . . . . . . . . . ventilation/perfusion

WBC . . . . . . . . white blood cells, white blood count